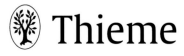

# Colorectal Tumors

## Atlas of Large Section Histopathology

Tibor Tot, MD
Associate Professor of Pathology
University of Uppsala School of Medicine
Head of Department of Pathology and Clinical Cytology
Central Hospital, Falun
Sweden

293 illustrations

Thieme
Stuttgart · New York

*Library of Congress Cataloging-in-Publication Data*

Tot, Tibor.
Histopathology of colorectal tumors / Tibor Tot.
    p. ; cm.
Includes bibliographical references and index.
ISBN 3-13-140591-0 (alk. paper) — ISBN 1-58890-384-2
(alk. paper)
1. Colon (Anatomy)—Cancer—Histopathology—Case studies.
2. Rectum—Cancer-Histopathology—Case studies.
[DNLM: 1. Colorectal Neoplasms—pathology—Case Reports.
WI 529 T717h 2005] I. Title.
RC280.C6T68 2005
616.99'434707—dc22

                        2005009276

**Important note:** Medicine is an ever-changing science undergoing continual development. Research and clinical experience are continually expanding our knowledge, in particular our knowledge of proper treatment and drug therapy. Insofar as this book mentions any dosage or application, readers may rest assured that the authors, editors, and publishers have made every effort to ensure that such references are in accordance with **the state of knowledge at the time of production of the book.**
Nevertheless, this does not involve, imply, or express any guarantee or responsibility on the part of the publishers in respect to any dosage instructions and forms of applications stated in the book. **Every user is requested to examine carefully** the manufacturers' leaflets accompanying each drug and to check, if necessary in consultation with a physician or specialist, whether the dosage schedules mentioned therein or the contraindications stated by the manufacturers differ from the statements made in the present book. Such examination is particularly important with drugs that are either rarely used or have been newly released on the market. Every dosage schedule or every form of application used is entirely at the user's own risk and responsibility. The authors and publishers request every user to report to the publishers any discrepancies or inaccuracies noticed. If errors in this work are found after publication, errata will be posted at www.thieme.com on the product description page.

Some of the product names, patents, and registered designs referred to in this book are in fact registered trademarks or proprietary names even though specific reference to this fact is not always made in the text. Therefore, the appearance of a name without designation as proprietary is not to be construed as a representation by the publisher that it is in the public domain.

© 2005 Georg Thieme Verlag,
Rüdigerstrasse 14, 70469 Stuttgart, Germany
http://www.thieme.de
Thieme New York, 333 Seventh Avenue,
New York, NY 10001 USA
http://www.thieme.com

Typesetting by primustype R. Hurler GmbH, Notzingen
Printed in Germany by Grammlich, Pliezhausen

ISBN 3-13-140591-0 (GTV)
ISBN 1-58890-384-2 (TNY)            1 2 3 4 5

# Contents

# Acknowledgement

To produce a high-quality large histological section is a complex and difficult task. The most important factor in this applied art is the skillful and ambitious laboratory technician. I wish to thank all my co-workers involved in producing large histological sections for the pleasure of looking at their artistic masterpieces and to dedicate this book to Britta Elborg, Britt-Marie Ericsson, Marie Högström, Evelyn Karlsson, Birgitta Norén, to Lena Arvidsson, Irene Bergman, Kajsa Engfeldt, Birgitta Lind, Ingegerd Lindquist, Anita Paulsson and their colleagues. I hope that the reader will share my appreciation.

# Introduction

Intestinal and, especially, colorectal diseases represent one of the most common medical problems of humankind, with colorectal carcinoma being one of the most frequently occurring malignancies in Europe and America (Parkin et al. 1992). General practitioners, gastroenterologists, oncologists, radiologists, surgeons, and nurses treat thousands of patients with intestinal diseases every day all over the world. The correct diagnosis is essential for administering the proper therapy. In spite of the rapid developments that have taken place in many fields of modern medical science, histopathology remains essential in making or confirming a diagnosis in a substantial proportion of intestinal diseases.

The attention of the medical community has gradually shifted from morphology towards molecules and genes, which has led to significant progress in many fields of modern medicine, pathology included. However, this shift also risks replacing knowledge about diseases with knowledge about numbers, expressed in a language made up of hardly understandable abbreviations. In addition, in the minds of many medical students and medical doctors, digital images generated by modern radiology have replaced the „gold standard" of autopsy findings. As a result, knowledge derived from advanced technology is gradually replacing knowledge that has been diligently collected over a period of hundreds of years. The danger of this process is that not only will information be lost, but, more importantly, it will be replaced with something less accurate. Physicians who regularly correlate their endoscopic and radiological images with pathoanatomical and histopathological findings may avoid this mistake. Unfortunately, in this era of unacceptably low autopsy rates, such a physician has less and less opportunity to do so.

Although it is hardly possible to offer equally valuable alternatives to information obtained from autopsy findings, pathologists must try to help clinicians in correlating clinical, radiological and endoscopic findings with morphology. Today, there are many different options that can be explored, such as clinical pathology conferences, telepathology and publishing macroscopic and histologic photographs digitally or on the World Wide Web.

In addition to the clinical picture, the macroscopic appearance of the colorectal mucosa and the nature of the lesions on it, as seen with an endoscope, represent the basis for clinical diagnosis. Endoscopists regularly take biopsies of the mucosa and/or endoscopically evident lesions for histopathological analysis in order to confirm the clinical diagnosis or to detect alterations not visible endoscopically. However, the histologic details cannot be directly compared with the endoscopic appearance of the lesions. For this reason, the pathology report most often provides descriptive information, which the endoscopist cannot directly connect to the image seen in vivo. Large histologic sections, by preserving the contiguity of the tissue in a representative transection of the bowel lesion, bridge the gap between the endoscopic and the histologic appearance. Projected as an overhead, the large section not only resembles the endoscopic findings but at the same time also magnifies them, allowing the clinician to analyze the relief and the details of the lesions on the gross and subgross levels. Placing the same large histologic section under the microscope, the pathologist can demonstrate the histo-

logic and cellular details behind the subgross findings. This makes large histologic sections an ideal approach to educating and training residents as well as specialists performing gastrointestinal endoscopy.

The advantages of using large histologic sections are not exclusively educational. This technique has been routinely used in our laboratory for every operative breast specimen since 1984, and convincing evidence about its suitability in routine diagnostic procedures has been collected. While the resolution of the cellular details are on the level of those obtained with the conventional small block technique, large histologic sections reveal much more useful information than derived from small section, since they usually include a representative transection of the entire tumor together with its environment and the circumferential surgical margins. This technique has proven to be more reliable in documenting the size of the tumor and the extent and distribution of the disease in the breast. It is also superior in demonstrating the multifocal nature of the tumor and intertumoral heterogeneity, compared to the traditional techniques of tissue sampling (Jackson et al. 1994; Tot et al. 2000). In fact, some prognostically important parameters of certain types of breast carcinoma can only be reliably assessed using large histologic sections (Tot 2003).

Surgery remains fundamental in treating patients with gastrointestinal tumors, and it is the best option for cure in patients with rectal cancer, provided that the procedure is radical. During the last two decades, a modified surgical intervention, called total mesorectal resection, has been introduced as a procedure of choice, since it has been shown to lower the rate of local recurrences from 30–40% to less than 10% (Heald and Ryall 1986; Leong 2003; Cecil et al. 2004). The procedure is based on removal of the tumor together with the mesorectal fat. Assessment of the radicality of surgical intervention has always been an important task of the pathologist. In the technique of total mesorectal resection, it has become increasingly important since 2 mm or more of free tissue in the circumferential margin may assure local control of the disease (Nagtegaal et al. 2002). By integrating the gross and subgross appearances with the details of the histologic examination, the technique of large-section histology is an ideal tool for assessing the circumferential margin in total mesorectal resection specimens. It may also influence the content of the histopathology report, which varies considerably from institution to institution (Wei et al. 2004).

With the support of our gastrointestinal surgeons, in 1997, it was decided to include large-section histology in the routine histologic work-up of total mesorectal resection specimens. Based on our experience regarding the advantages of including this technique in the pathology work-up and in demonstrating and interpreting the findings in clinical conferences, the use of large-section histology was soon widened to every operated case of colorectal neoplasm and to some non-neoplastic intestinal lesions. During the last 7 years, almost 2000 cases of colorectal carcinoma and other intestinal lesions have been documented on large histologic sections, a collection that represents the basis for the present atlas.

Proper staging of colorectal carcinomas is essential for treatment and prognosis. The most widely used staging systems are the Dukes' classification (Dukes 1940) and the TNM classification (AJCC cancer staging handbook. TNM classification of malignant tumors, 6th edn. 2002). Despite the numerous attempts to modify the Dukes system, it has remained simple and easy to apply, although somewhat limited in its ability to stratify patients for proper therapy. The TNM classification system, by contrast, offers a more sensitive prognostic categorization due to the larger number of combinations of parameters for describing both the primary tumor and the presence or absence of metastasis in the examined lymph nodes or distant organs. However, new editions of the TNM system have become increasingly complicated and difficult to reproducibly apply. Large histologic sections, by showing the deepest level of invasion of the primary tumor together with the peritumoral tissue, which may contain isolated tumor foci and several lymph nodes, can help in proper tumor classification and staging. This technique brings the so-called pTNM (pathological TNM classification), based on histologic parameters, much closer to the clinical TNM classification. Thus, in this atlas, the term pTNM is not used.

Recent advances in modern radiology have resulted in more detailed imaging of the colorectum (Koh et al 2004). So-called virtual endoscopy may revolutionize gastroenterology as it offers a non-invasive method as an alternative to endoscopy. The technique is based on computer-tomography-produced images of horizontal transections of the bowel wall at different levels. As this approach is identical to that offered by the histopathologic technique of large sections, described in this atlas, it opens the way to new, previously unexplored perspectives in radiopathological correlation of intestinal lesions. Testing the accuracy of this new radiological method is obligatory, and large sections represent the ideal basis for correlation.

Although large histologic sections provide an advantageous alternative to the conventional small block technique, it is infrequently used in routine pathology laboratories. Many pathologists have criticized the technique of large histologic sections as being too expensive, unacceptably prolonging the technical procedure, causing problems in archiving of the slides, and adding nothing more than obtained with the traditional method of tissue sampling. However, our surgeons, gastroenterologists, oncologists, radiologists, pathologists, residents, medical students, and technicians, including those who have been more or less regularly involved in producing and interpreting large histologic sections and correlating them with their own clinical findings, as well as those who have only sporadically seen such sections, are enthusiastic. The usual feedback I get from them is that the information obtained from viewing large histologic slides has positively influenced their everyday practice. Several of them suggested that I share some of the large-section images of colorectal tumors with a wider professional audience. Thus, this atlas is as much a result of their support as of my own efforts.

# 1 Adenomas

## Case 1.1 Villous Adenoma of the Rectum

**Patient data:** 63-year-old woman presenting with rectal bleeding. Endoscopically, a large, broad-based, soft and exophytic tumor was seen in her rectum, diagnosed on preoperative biopsy as adenoma.

**Surgical treatment:** Rectosigmoidal resection, no preoperative irradiation.

**Specimen:** 35-cm-long rectosigmoideum with an 8 × 6-cm soft exophytic tumor, 3 cm from the distal margin.

**Histopathologic diagnosis:** Villous adenoma of the rectum with moderate dysplasia. No signs of severe dysplasia or invasion.

**Follow-up:** 81 months, without signs of disease recurrence.

Villous adenoma of the rectum is often a large non-pedunculated tumor, covering the rectal mucosa over an area of several centimeters. Endoscopic biopsies usually reach only the superficial part of the tumor, the delicate long villous structures covered by dysplastic epithelium. The large histologic section (Fig. 1.1) also demonstrates the intact lamina muscularis mucosae: no signs of invasion are present. It is easy to compare the structures of the normal bowel wall (indicated by the red arrow in the schematic image, Fig. 1.1 d) to the structures of the adenoma (the left side of the image, green arrows in Fig. 1.1 d). Adenomas exhibit a dysplastic epithelium. The transition from normal to dysplastic epithelium is illustrated in Figure 1.1 a (corresponding to the area marked with a red rectangle in Fig. 1.1 d). Figure 1.1 b represents a microscopic image of the delicate villous structures of the adenoma (corresponding to the blue rectangle in Fig. 1.1 d). Figure 1.1 c is a magnified detail of Figure 1.1 b, illustrating the moderately dysplastic epithelium of this adenoma exhibiting elongated, stratified and crowded cell nuclei and a reduced number of goblet cells.

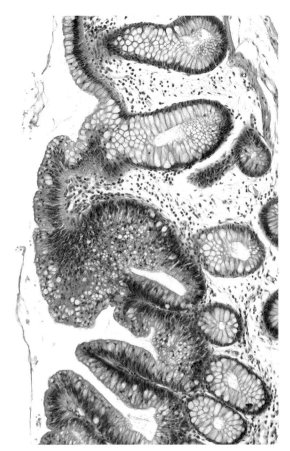

Fig. 1.**1 a**

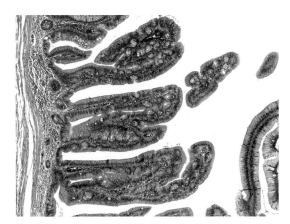

Fig. 1.**1 b**

### Practical points

- Villous adenomas are usually non-pedunculated, soft tumors covering a large area of the surface of the bowel wall. Large histologic sections are needed to visualize the entire lesion in one transection.
- The large histologic section is an ideal tool for assessing and demonstrating invasive tumor foci in such a large lesion, as these can be easily missed during the macroscopic examination and sampling of standard small blocks.

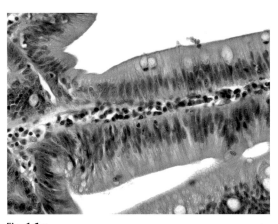

Fig. 1.**1 c**

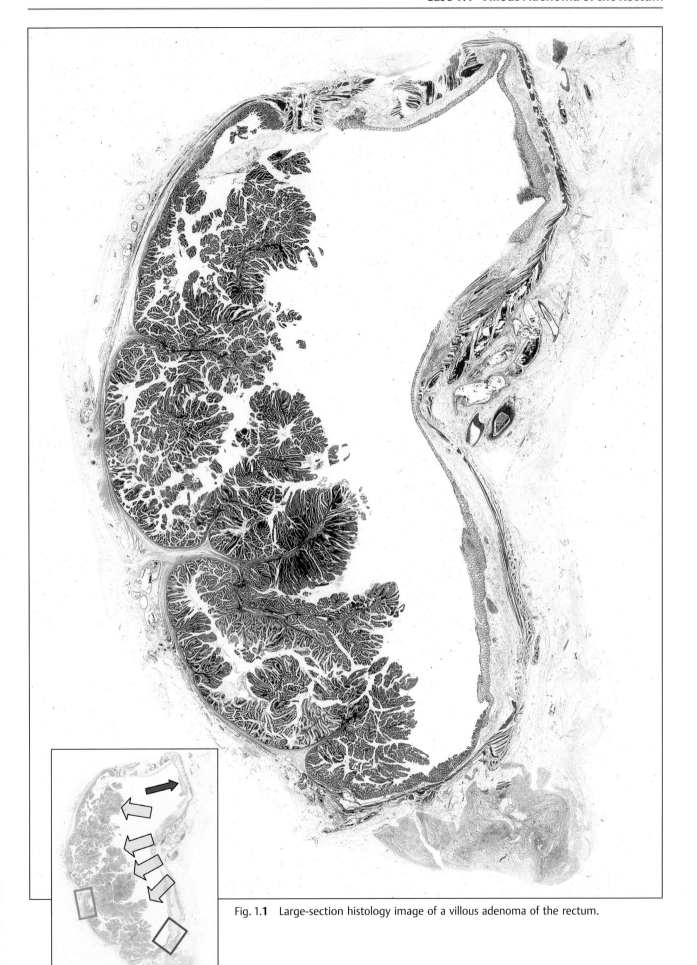

Fig. 1.**1** Large-section histology image of a villous adenoma of the rectum.

Fig. 1.**1 d** Schematic guide to the morphologic details in the large section in Fig. 1.**1**.

## Case 1.2 Villous Adenoma of the Rectum

**Patient data:** 84-year-old woman with intermittent rectal bleeding and a long history of recurrent adenomas in her rectum.

**Surgical treatment:** Rectosigmoidal resection, no pre-operative irradiation.

**Specimen:** 33-cm-long rectosigmoideum with a 9-cm segment containing a circumferential exophytic tumor, 6 cm from the distal margin.

**Histopathologic diagnosis:** Villous adenoma of the rectum with low-grade, partly moderate dysplasia. No signs of invasion.

**Follow-up:** 6 months, without signs of disease recurrence.

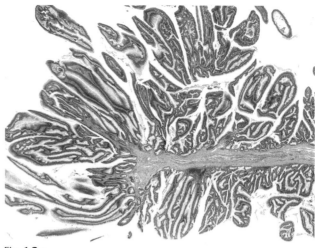

Fig. 1.2 a

The large section in Figure 1.2 demonstrates another case of villous adenoma, which covers the entire circumference of the inner surface of the rectum. No signs of invasion are seen. The architecture of villous adenomas is complex, as they consist of primary finger-like processes extending outward from the bowel wall and containing fibromuscular stroma (indicated with blue arrows in Fig. 1.2 c). Secondary finger-like processes, consisting of loose fibrous stroma with delicate vasculature and a surface covered by dysplastic epithelium, cover these structures. Figure 1.2 a, b illustrate the complexity of these structures (corresponding to the red rectangle in the schematic image, Fig. 1.2 c).

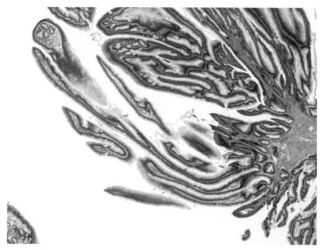

Fig. 1.2 b

**Practical points**

- Villous adenomas may cover large areas of the entire circumference of the bowel wall. Large histologic sections are needed to visualize the entire lesion in one transection.
- Large histologic sections are also an ideal tool for analyzing the subgross architecture of complex lesions like adenomas.

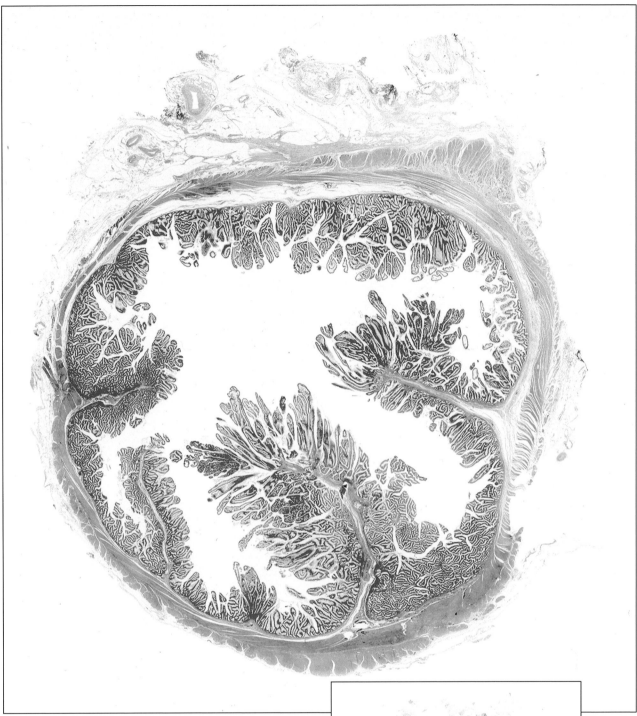

Fig. 1.**2**  Large-section histology image of a villous adenoma of the rectum.

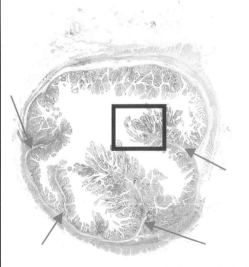

Fig. 1.**2c**  Schematic guide to the morphologic details in the large section in Fig. 1.**2**.

## Case 1.3 Villous Adenoma of the Colon

**Patient data:** 55-year-old male examined for weight loss. Colonoscopy detected a polypoid lesion in the sigmoid colon, diagnosed as adenoma on preoperative biopsy.
**Surgical treatment:** Sigmoidal resection, no preoperative irradiation.
**Specimen:** 15-cm-long segment of the sigmoid colon containing a 3 × 3-cm exophytic tumor, 3 cm from the distal margin.
**Histopathologic diagnosis:** Villous adenoma with moderate dysplasia. No signs of invasion.
**Follow-up:** 31 months, no signs of disease recurrence. The patient developed prostate cancer 12 months after the sigmoideum resection.

The large section (Fig. 1.3) in the present case contains a transection of a villous adenoma of the sigmoid colon with long villous structures (magnified in Fig. 1.3 a; the corresponding area is indicated by the yellow rectangle in Fig. 1.3 d). Structures from the mesocolon are also seen in the same large section: a lymph node (indicated by the green arrow in Fig. 1.3 d and magnified in Fig. 1.3 b) and mesenterial blood vessels (indicated by the red rectangle in Fig. 1.3 d and magnified in Fig. 1.3 c). The large sections regularly include structures from the mesocolon, which is advantageous when assessing the extent of tumor growth.

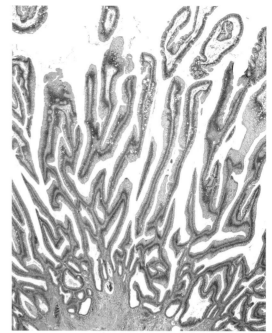

Fig. 1.**3 a**

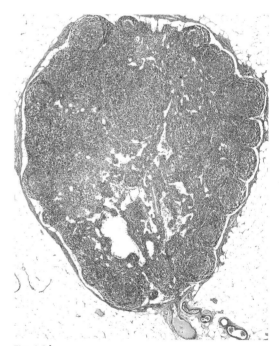

Fig. 1.**3 b**

### Practical points

- Large histologic sections include a continuous tissue containing a transection of the bowel wall, a transection of the pathologic lesion(s), and a part of the mesenterial/periintestinal tissue. This non-fragmented image allows assessment of the relation of the lesion(s) to the surrounding structures.
- Lymph nodes and vascular structures, together with the intestinal lesion(s), can easily be analyzed in the large sections.

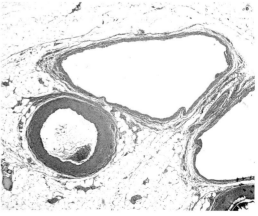

Fig. 1.**3 c**

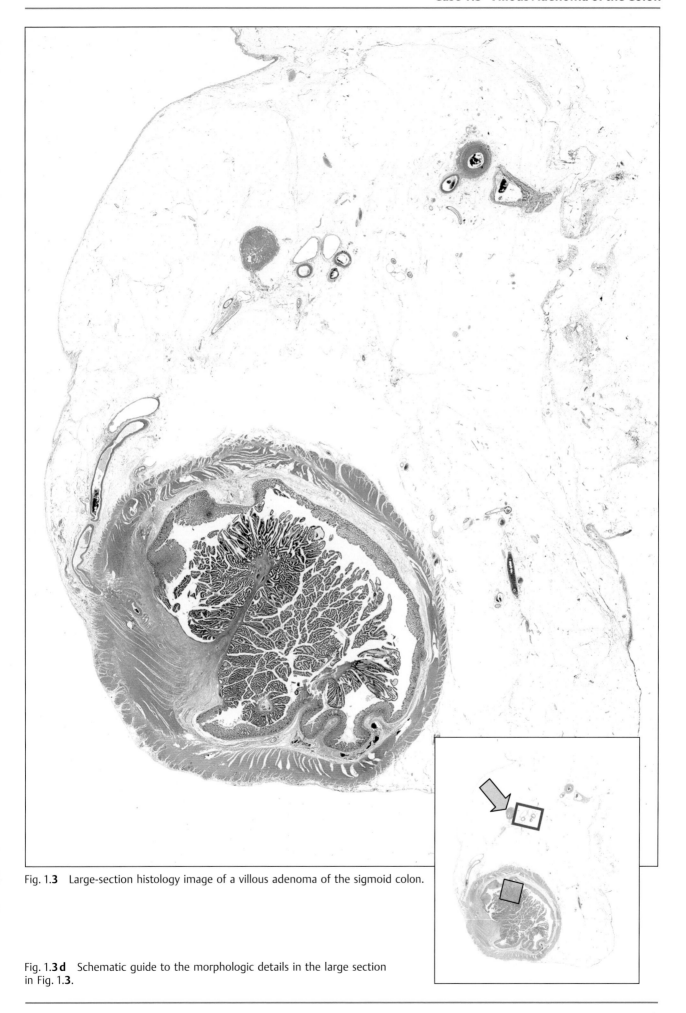

Fig. 1.**3** Large-section histology image of a villous adenoma of the sigmoid colon.

Fig. 1.**3 d** Schematic guide to the morphologic details in the large section in Fig. 1.**3**.

## Case 1.4 Mucinous Carcinoma of the Rectum That Developed in a Villous Adenoma

**Patient data:** 88-year-old woman presenting with rectal bleeding. Endoscopically, an exophytic lesion was seen in her rectum. The preoperative endoscopic biopsy contained exclusively structures of adenoma.

**Surgical treatment:** Rectosigmoidal resection, no preoperative irradiation.

**Specimen:** 20-cm-long rectosigmoideum with a 6 × 5-cm exophytic tumor, 5 cm from the distal margin.

**Histopathologic diagnosis:** Mucinous carcinoma, low grade, infiltrating in but not beyond the lamina muscularis propria, 23 lymph nodes without signs of metastasis, radical excision, mesorectal margin 20 mm.

**TNM stage:** I (T2N0M0), Dukes A.

**Follow-up:** 36 months, without signs of disease recurrence.

Mucinous carcinoma may develop in villous adenomas. The large histologic section in Figure 1.4 demonstrates not only the mucinous carcinoma (green-colored area in the schematic image, Fig. 1.4c), but also the structures of the rests of the adenoma (orange arrows) as well as their relation to the cancer. To obtain a representative endoscopic biopsy, one has to reach the invasive part of the tumor, which is partly covered by the villous structures of the adenoma. Figure 1.4a, a microscopic magnification of the area indicated by the white rectangle in Figure 1.4c, shows the interface of the villous adenoma and the mucinous carcinoma. The large section offers proper documentation of the level of tumor invasion and, at the same time, reliably demonstrates the circumferential margin, including the mesorectal surgical resection margin. The mesorectal resection margin is easily assessed and its distance to the deepest invasive tumor structures is easy to measure, as indicated by the red double arrow in Figure 1.4c. The deepest level of invasion is indicated by the yellow rectangle in Figure 1.4c and is microscopically magnified in Figure 1.4b. Note also the four small reactive lymph nodes in the fatty tissue (encircled in Fig. 1.4c).

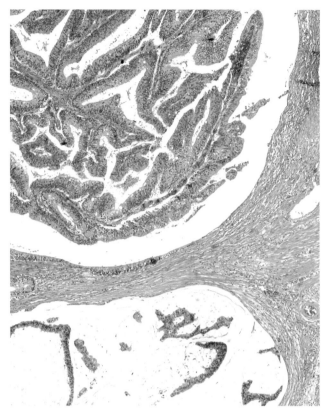

Fig. 1.4a

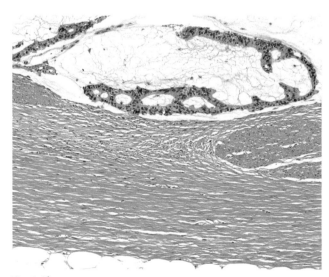

Fig. 1.4b

### Practical points

- In order to obtain a representative biopsy, the endoscopist has to reach the invasive cancer, which is often covered by the rests of the adenoma.
- Taken in the plane of the deepest invasion, the large histologic sections reliably document the level of tumor growth.
- Large histologic sections are an ideal tool for assessing and demonstrating the circumferential surgical margin and its relation to the invasive tumor.

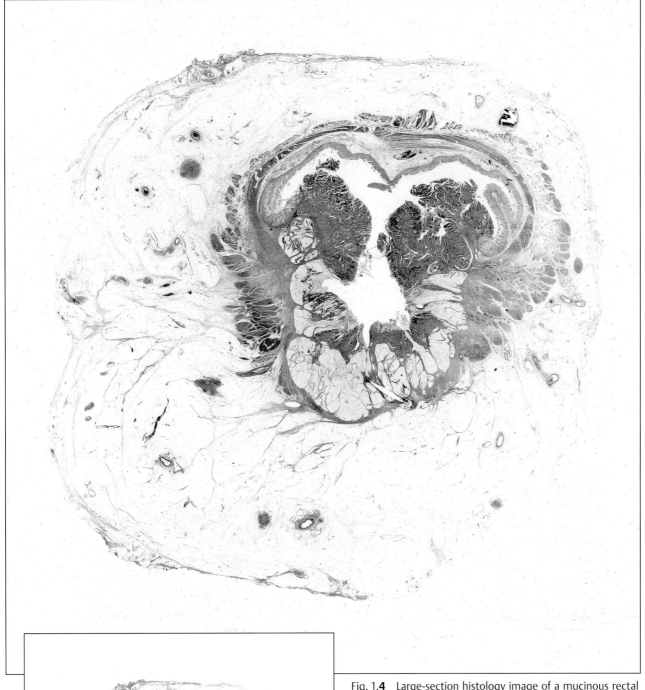

Fig. 1.**4**   Large-section histology image of a mucinous rectal carcinoma that developed in a villous adenoma.

Fig. 1.**4c**   Schematic guide to the morphologic details in the large section in Fig. 1.**4**.

## Case 1.5 Rectal Carcinoma That Developed in a Villous Adenoma

**Patient data:** 78-year-old man presenting with rectal bleeding. Endoscopically, a large exophytic tumor was seen in his rectum. The preoperative biopsy contained only structures of an adenoma with high-grade dysplasia.
**Surgical treatment:** Mesorectal resection, no preoperative irradiation.
**Specimen:** 20-cm-long rectum with a 7 × 4-cm exophytic tumor, 10 cm from the distal margin.
**Histopathologic diagnosis:** Well- differentiated infiltrating adenocarcinoma, partly with mucinous differentiation, 7 of 8 examined lymph nodes containing metastasis. Radical excision, mesorectal margin 15 mm.
**TNM stage:** IIIc (T2N2M0), Dukes C.
**Follow-up:** 29 months, without signs of disease recurrence.

The partly mucinous rectal carcinoma demonstrated in the large histologic section in Figure 1.5 has developed in a villous adenoma. The deepest level of invasion in the bowel wall (corresponding to the area of the green rectangle in the schematic image, Fig. 1.5 d) is microscopically magnified in Figure 1.5 a. Although the cancer was relatively small and well differentiated, it metastasized to the regional lymph nodes, one of which was present in the large section and is indicated by the blue arrow in Figure 1.5. The lymph node metastasis is microscopically magnified in Figure 1.5 b. The cancer also infiltrated the tissue around the blood vessels of the mesocolon in the form of isolated invasive tumor foci, as demonstrated in Figure 1.5 c (corresponding to the encircled area in Fig. 1.5 d). Obtaining an endoscopic biopsy representing the invasive part of the lesion may be a very difficult task in such a case.

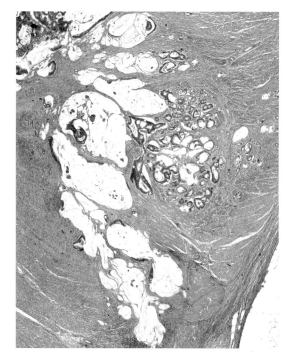

Fig. 1.5 a

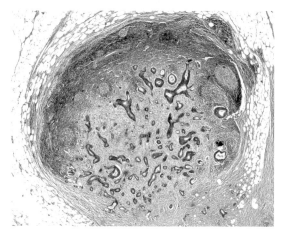

Fig. 1.5 b

### Practical points

- In order to obtain a representative biopsy, the endoscopist has to reach the invasive cancer, which is often covered by the rests of the adenoma.
- By including a part of the mesorectal tissue that is continuous with the transection of the rectum, the large histologic section facilitates assessment of perirectal tumor dissemination in relation to the primary tumor.

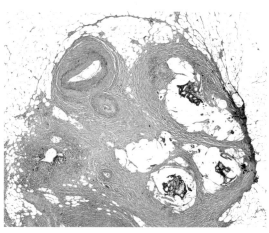

Fig. 1.5 c

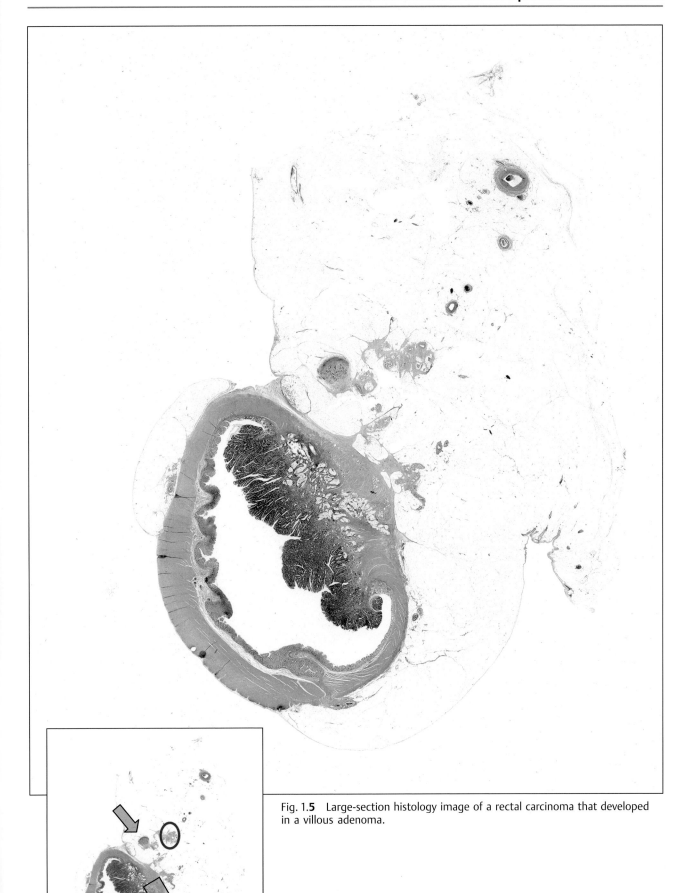

**Fig. 1.5**  Large-section histology image of a rectal carcinoma that developed in a villous adenoma.

**Fig. 1.5 d**  Schematic guide to the morphologic details in the large section in Fig. 1.**5**.

## Case 1.6 Tubulovillous Adenoma of the Cecum

**Patient data:** 81-year-old man presenting with bloody diarrhea. Endoscopically, two separate polypoid lesions were seen, one in the colon ascendens and the other in the cecum.
**Surgical treatment:** Right hemicolectomy.
**Specimen:** 40-cm-long part of the colon with a 3 × 3-cm exophytic tumor 18 cm from the distal margin and, 10 cm from it, a separate polypoid lesion in the cecum.
**Histopathologic diagnosis:** Infiltrating adenocarcinoma, partly with signet-ring cell differentiation, developed in an adenoma. No metastasis in 17 examined lymph nodes. Radical excision. A separate tubulovillous adenoma with moderate dysplasia in the cecum.
**TNM stage:** I (T2N0M0), Dukes A.
**Follow-up:** Died of leukemia 8 months later.

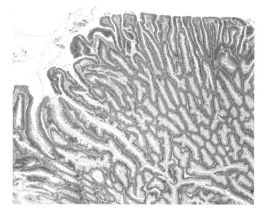

Fig. 1.**6a**

This patient had a carcinoma in his colon ascendens (not presented here) and an additional separate large polypoid lesion in his cecum. The histology of the lesion presented in Figure 1.**6** shows the structures of a tubulovillous adenoma, partly with finger-like excrescences, but mainly with tubular gland-like spaces (magnified in Fig. 1.**6a**, corresponding to the area marked with the blue arrow in the schematic image, Fig. 1.**6e**). The difference between the normal mucosa (lower-left part of the image) and the dysplastic epithelium of the adenoma (upper-right part of the image) is well seen in Figure 1.**6b**, which represents a histologic magnification of the area of the green rectangle in Figure 1.**6e**. The large-section image (Fig. 1.**6**) demonstrates well that the lesion has a branching fibrous core, free of tumor structures; no signs of invasion could be evidenced. Details of the fibrous core are magnified in Figure 1.**6c, d** (corresponding to the orange circle and to the yellow rectangle in Fig. 1.**6e**, respectively). This adenoma is somewhat pedunculated, exhibiting a relatively narrow stalk (as compared to the tumor in the patient described in Case 1.7).

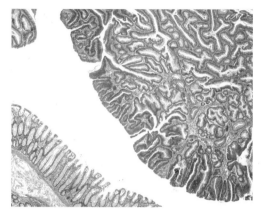

Fig. 1.**6b**

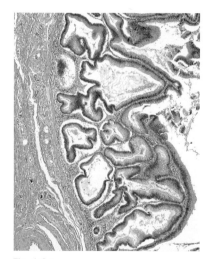

Fig. 1.**6c**

### Practical points

- As a large histologic section can demonstrate a transection of an entire adenoma, it allows assessment of both a contiguous tissue of the stromal core and the epithelial structures. Detailed analysis of the stroma is especially important in larger adenomas, as malignant transformation and invasion occur more frequently at these sites.

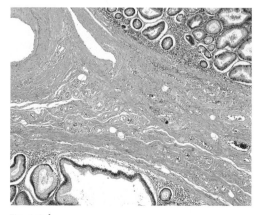

Fig. 1.**6d**

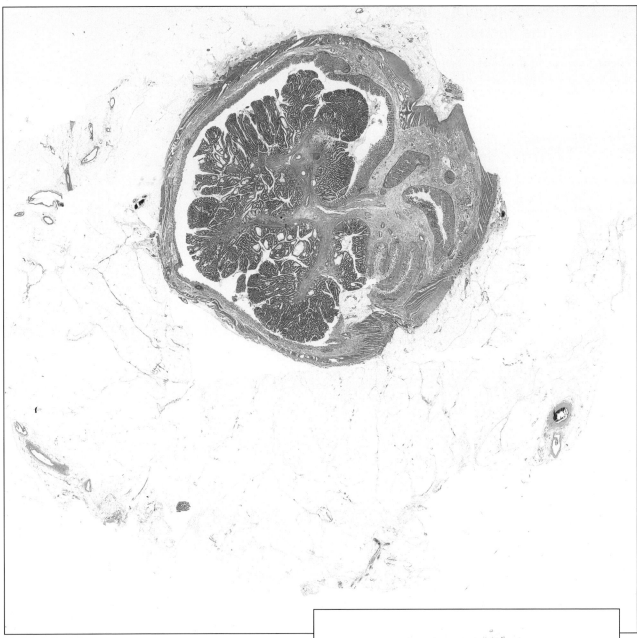

Fig. 1.**6**   Large-section histology image of a tubulovillous adenoma of the cecum.

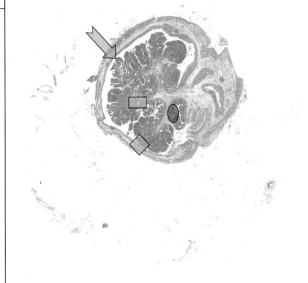

Fig. 1.**6 e**   Schematic guide to the morphologic details in the large section in Fig. 1.**6**.

## Case 1.7 Tubulovillous Adenoma of the Rectum

**Patient data:** 82-year-old man with a history of rectal bleeding over several years. Endoscopically, a large broad-based polypoid mass was seen in his rectum. Although the preoperative histologic diagnosis was adenoma, the patient underwent surgery on the basis of the clinical and endoscopic picture.

**Surgical treatment:** Mesorectal resection, no preoperative irradiation.

**Specimen:** 30-cm-long rectosigmoideum with a 4 × 3-cm polypoid lesion, 4 cm from the distal margin.

**Histopathologic diagnosis:** Tubulovillous adenoma of the rectum with moderate to severe dysplasia. No signs of invasion.

**Follow-up:** 15 months, without signs of disease recurrence.

The large histologic section in this case (Fig. 1.**7**) demonstrates an adenoma with a broad base containing large blood vessels (indicated with an arrow in the schematic image, Fig. 1.**7 a**). The stroma is free of tumor structures; no signs of infiltration are seen. Broad-based adenomas, especially if larger, may give an impression of malignancy when seen endoscopically. Compared to the adenoma discussed in the previous case (Case 1.6, a pedunculated adenoma with a narrow, delicate stalk), this adenoma is much more sessile, covering a larger area of the intestinal surface.

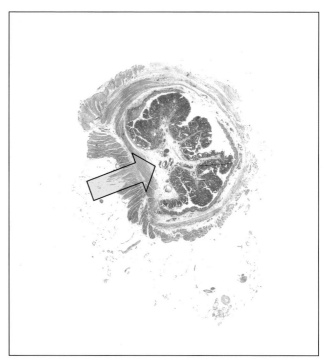

Fig. 1.**7 a**  Schematic guide to the morphologic details in the large section in Fig. 1.**7**.

### Practical points

- When seen endoscopically, large sessile adenomas may give a false impression of malignancy.
- Large histologic sections represent an ideal tool for assessing such lesions, as the entire adenoma, with its dysplastic epithelium and broad stalk, together with the surrounding tissue, can be imaged.

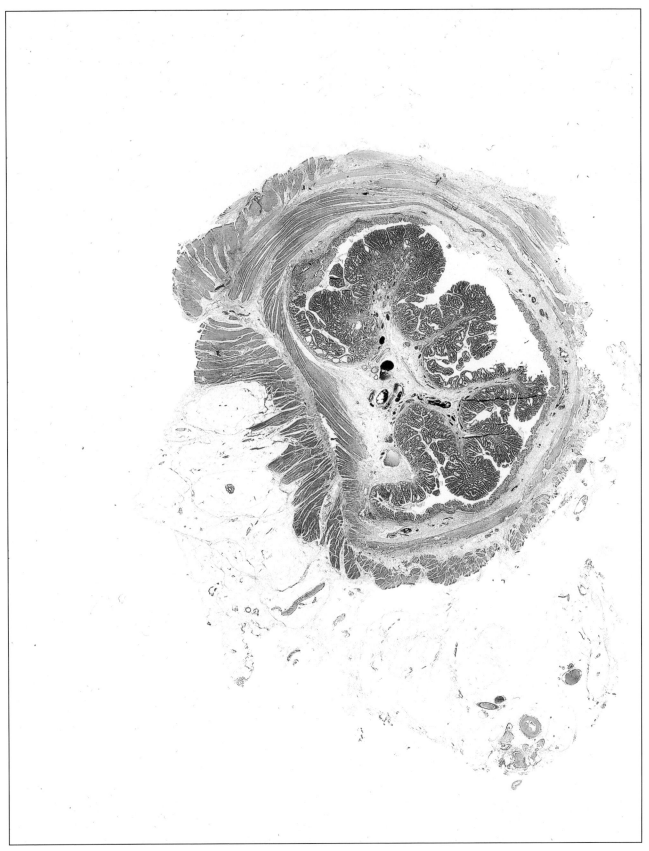

Fig. 1.**7** Large-section histology image of a tubulovillous adenoma of the rectum.

## Case 1.8 Tubulovillous Adenoma of the Colon with Severe Dysplasia

**Patient data:** 62-year-old woman presenting with bloody stools. Endoscopically, a pedunculated polypoid lesion was seen in the sigmoideum. Preoperative histologic examination of the endoscopic biopsies revealed structures of adenoma with severe dysplasia.
**Surgical treatment:** Sigmoidal resection.
**Specimen:** 14-cm-long segment of the large bowel with a 4 × 2-cm polypoid lesion 3 cm from the distal margin.
**Histopathologic diagnosis:** Tubulovillous adenoma with moderate to severe dysplasia. No signs of invasion.
**Follow-up:** 26 months, no signs of disease recurrence.

The large histologic section in this case demonstrates a pedunculated tubulovillous adenoma of the colon (Fig. 1.**8**). The mucosa surrounding the adenoma exhibited hyperplastic changes. The interface of the adenomatous and hyperplastic structures is demonstrated in Figure 1.**8a** (corresponding to the area marked with the green arrow in Fig. 1.**8d**). The surface of the adenoma contained a small area of granulation tissue at the site of preoperative endoscopic biopsy (magnified in Fig. 1.**8b**, corresponding to the area of the red arrow in Fig. 1.**8d**). The delicate branching stroma of the tumor is well demonstrated in the large section. No signs of invasion could be detected, but focally the tumor contained areas of severe dysplasia. One of these foci is marked with the yellow rectangle in Figure 1.**8d** and is microscopically magnified in Figure 1.**8c**.

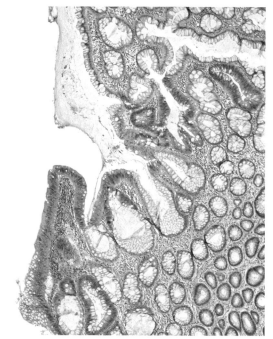

Fig. 1.**8a**

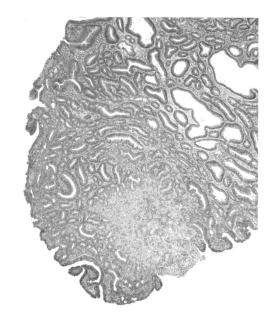

Fig. 1.**8b**

### Practical points

As a large histologic section may include a transection of the entire adenoma, it shows the contiguous tissue of the stromal core and the epithelial structures. Detailed analysis of the epithelium is important to detect severe dysplasia and malignant transformation.

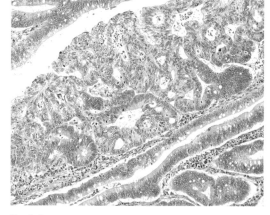

Fig. 1.**8c**

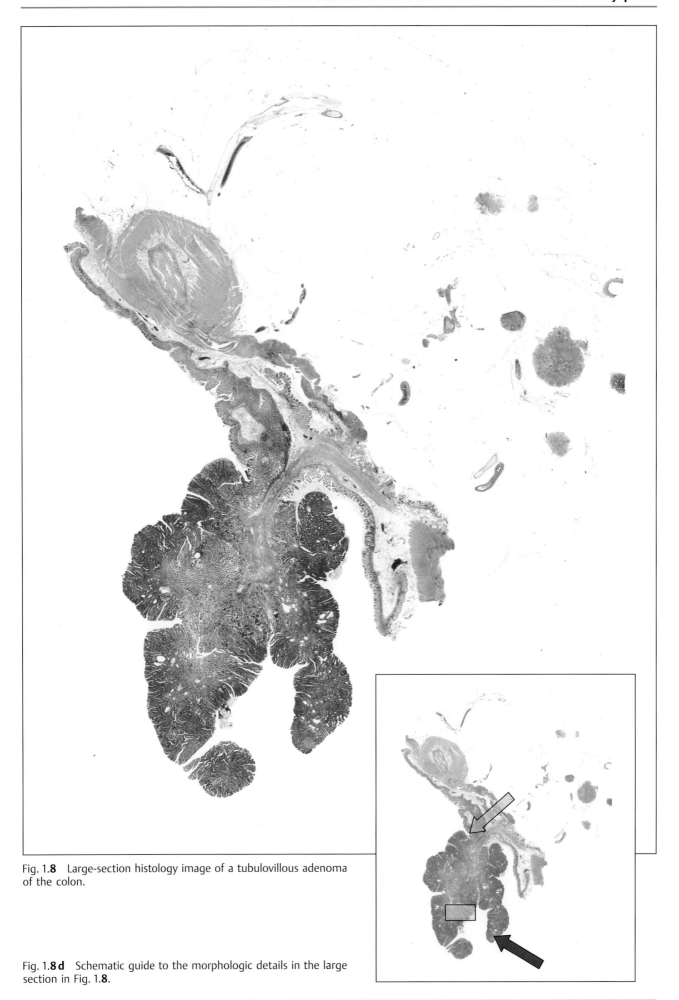

Fig. 1.8  Large-section histology image of a tubulovillous adenoma of the colon.

Fig. 1.8 d  Schematic guide to the morphologic details in the large section in Fig. 1.8.

## Case 1.9 Tubulovillous Adenoma Associated with Invasive Carcinoma

**Patient data:** 75-year-old woman presenting with anemia. Endoscopically, a pedunculated polypoid lesion and a separate ulcerated tumor were seen at the border between the sigmoideum and rectum. Preoperative histologic examination of the endoscopic biopsies (from the ulcerated tumor) revealed invasive carcinoma.
**Surgical treatment:** Rectosigmoidal resection, no preoperative irradiation.
**Specimen:** 20-cm-long segment of the large bowel with a 1-cm polypoid lesion and a 4 × 3-cm ulcerated tumor, 14 cm from the distal margin.
**Histopathologic diagnosis:** Tubulovillous adenoma with moderate dysplasia. Moderately differentiated invasive adenocarcinoma growing in but not penetrating the lamina muscularis propria. Two of the 12 examined lymph nodes contained metastasis.
**TNM stage:** IIIa(T2N1M0), Dukes C.
**Follow-up:** 39 months, no signs of disease recurrence.

This large histologic section (Fig. 1.**9**) was taken through an invasive carcinoma, seen on the right side of the image (the red-colored area on the schematic image, Fig. 1.**9 c**), and also includes a transection of a separate pedunculated tubulovillous adenoma, seen on the left side of the image (marked with the green arrow in Fig. 1.**9 c**). The large section demonstrates the level of tumoral invasion within the lamina muscularis propria (magnified in Fig. 1.**9 a**, corresponding to the area of the blue rectangle in Fig. 1.**9 c**). The large histologic section also showed some mesenterial lymph nodes, one of them (marked with the orange rectangle in Fig. 1.**9 c** and microscopically magnified in Fig. 1.**9 b**) containing metastasis.

**Practical points**

- Large histologic section may include several different lesions, allowing the interrelation of these lesions to be analyzed.
- Inclusion of the mesorectal/mesocolic lymph nodes is a further advantage of large sections, as it may assist the pathologist in proper staging of the tumor.

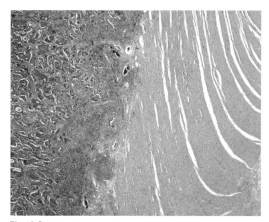

Fig. 1.**9 a**

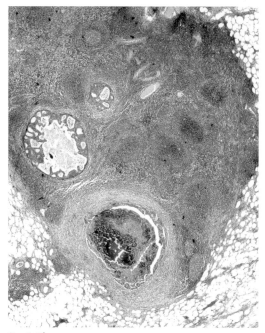

Fig. 1.**9 b**

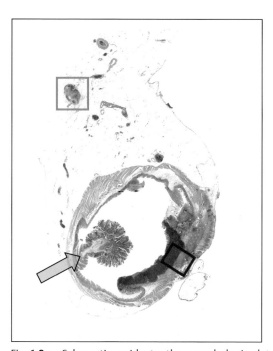

Fig. 1.**9 c** Schematic guide to the morphologic details in the large section in Fig. 1.**9**.

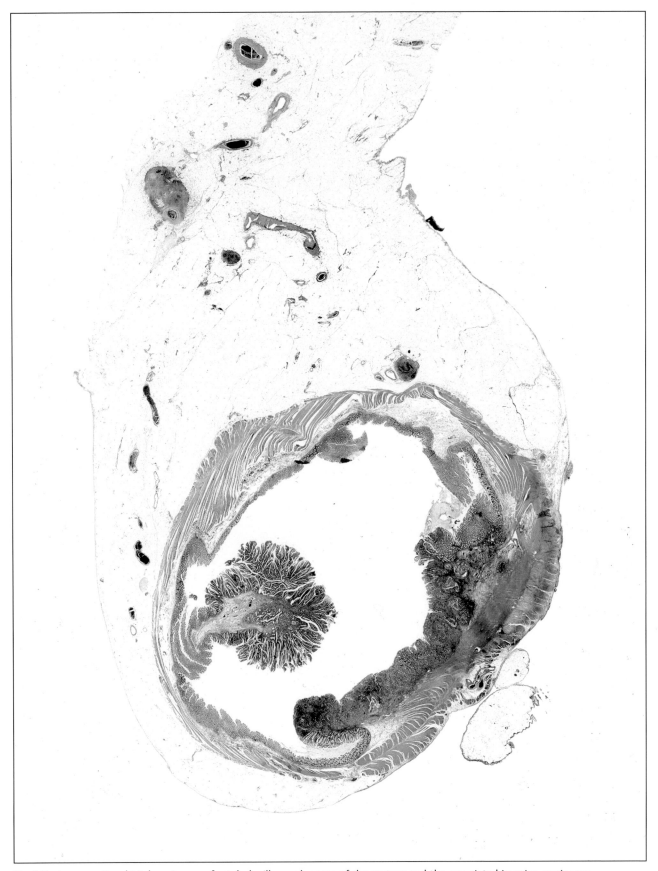

Fig. 1.**9**   Large-section histology image of a tubulovillous adenoma of the rectum and the associated invasive carcinoma.

## Case 1.10 Hamartomatous Polyposis of the Small Intestine (Peutz–Jeghers Syndrome)

**Patient data:** 40-year-old woman with Peutz–Jeghers syndrome operated on for acute intestinal obstruction.
**Surgical treatment:** Short-segment jejunal resection.
**Specimen:** 10-cm-long segment of the small bowel with approximately 20 pedunculated polyps unevenly distributed within the specimen.
**Histopathologic diagnosis:** Hamartomatous polyposis typical of Peutz–Jeghers syndrome. No malignancy.
**Follow-up:** 9 months, with an episode of upper gastrointestinal bleeding when multiple gastric and duodenal polyps were examined endoscopically; these were diagnosed at biopsy as Peutz–Jeghers polyps.

The large histologic section in Figure 1.**10** demonstrates multiple hamartomatous polyps in the small intestine of a patient with Peutz–Jeghers syndrome. As the presence of multiple polyps may complicate preparation of the specimen, it was difficult to obtain a non-fragmented large-section slice. The presented level of transection contains at least ten individual pedunculated polyps (some of them marked with green circles in Fig. 1.**10 d**). One of the polyps (marked with the red rectangle in Fig. 1.**10 d**) is microscopically magnified in Figure 1.**10 a**. Further magnification of the histological details in Figure 1.**10 a** is provided in Figure 1.**10 b**, **c**. The abnormal arborizing smooth-muscle bundles in the stroma are typical of polyps in Peutz–Jeghers syndrome. The crypts are irregular and somewhat dilated. Villous and papillary projections are seen on the surface of these polyps. The cells of the epithelium correspond to the elements of the normal small bowel. These polyps are different from multiple adenomas as they lack epithelial dysplasia. Several polypous lesions may mimic adenomas. As adenomatous polyposis is a well-recognized high-risk precancerous condition, it is important to histologically delineate this condition from macroscopically similar other polyposes. See also Cases 5.4 and 5.5.

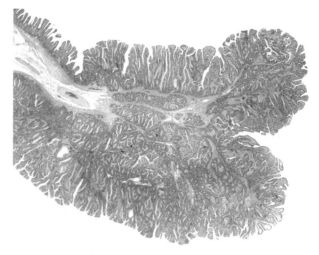

Fig. 1.**10 a**

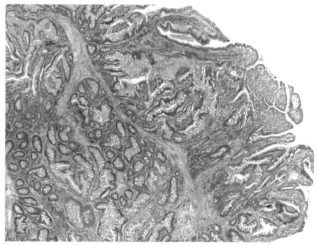

Fig. 1.**10 b**

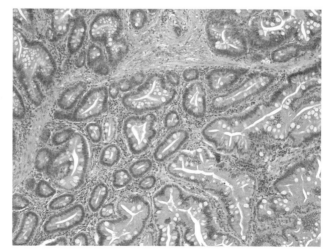

Fig. 1.**10 c**

### Practical points

- As the large histologic section may include several lesions, it facilitates proper histologic work-up of different polyposes.
- Histologic analysis of large sections has the advantage of including a large number of individual lesions on a single slide.

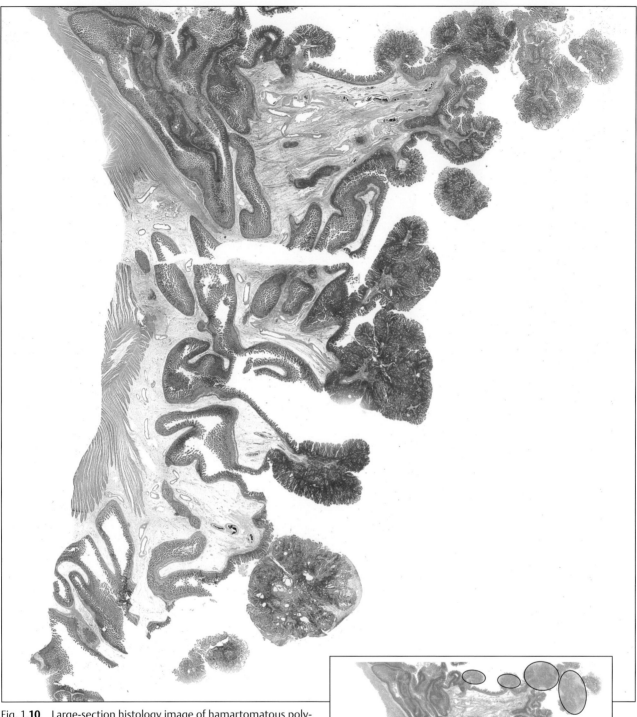

Fig. 1.**10** Large-section histology image of hamartomatous polyposis of the small intestine (in Peutz–Jeghers syndrome).

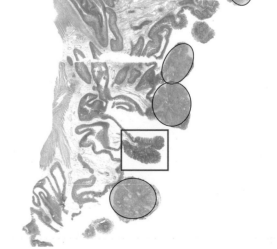

Fig. 1.**10 d** Schematic guide to the morphologic details in the large section in Fig. 1.**10**.

# 2 Early Colorectal Cancer

## Case 2.1 Early Carcinoma of the Rectum

**Patient data:** 65-year-old woman with rectal pain. Endoscopically, a small suspicious lesion was found 7 cm from the anus. A preoperative diagnosis of invasive carcinoma was made on endoscopic biopsy.

**Surgical treatment:** Mesorectal resection, no preoperative irradiation.

**Specimen:** 22-cm-long rectum with an exophytic tumor 15 mm in diameter, 1 cm from the distal margin.

**Histopathologic diagnosis:** Moderately differentiated rectal adenocarcinoma infiltrating into the submucosa and reaching the inner layer of the lamina muscularis propria, 13 lymph nodes without signs of metastasis, radical excision, mesorectal margin 22 mm.

**TNM stage:** I (T2N0M0), Dukes A.

**Follow-up:** 12 months, no signs of disease recurrence.

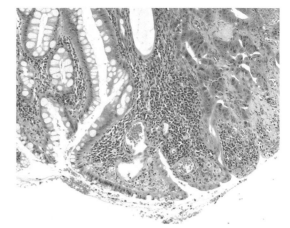

Fig. 2.**1a**

The level of the deepest invasion of the tumor and the presence or absence of metastasis are the most important prognostic factors in colorectal cancer. Tumors without metastasis and confined to the bowel wall (corresponding to stage A in Dukes' system or to one of the categories T1 or T2 in the TNM classification) have a good prognosis and may be designated as early colorectal cancer. Thus, proper assessment of the deepest level of tumoral invasion is crucial for adequate staging of the disease. The early rectal cancer in the presented case infiltrated only the submucosa of the rectum. As demonstrated in Figure 2.**1**, the tumor (corresponding to the red-colored area in the schematic image, Fig. 2.**1d**) just touched the inner muscular layer while the rest of the lamina muscularis propria remained intact. The abrupt transition from normal mucosa to neoplastic tissue, shown in Figure 2.**1a** (a microscopic magnification of the area of the red rectangle in Fig. 2.**1d**), indicates that this tumor may have developed without a precancerous stage of adenoma. The deepest level of infiltration (corresponding to the yellow rectangle in Fig. 2.**1d**) is microscopically magnified in Figure 2.**1b**. Further magnification of the same structures is seen in Figure 2.**1c**. As marked with the green colored circles in the schematic image, the large section contained four perirectal lymph nodes, which were free of metastasis. A continuous circumferential surgical margin (green-lined periphery of the specimen in Fig. 2.**1d**) is also shown; its distance to the nearest level of invasion is easy to assess.

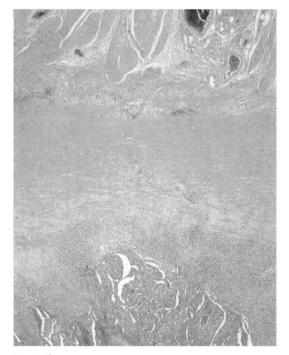

Fig. 2.**1b**

### Practical points

- Taken in the plane of the deepest invasion, the large histologic section provides reliable medical documentation of the level of primary tumor growth.
- Large histologic sections are an ideal tool for assessing and demonstrating the circumferential surgical margin and its relation to the invasive cancer.

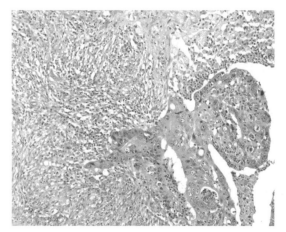

Fig. 2.**1c**

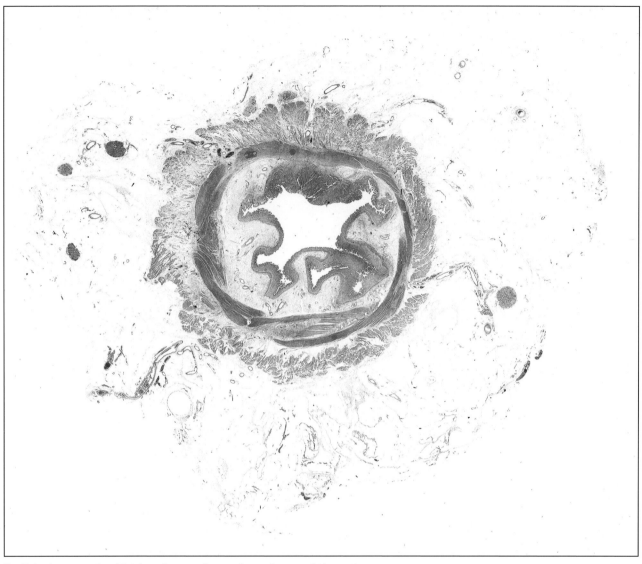

Fig. 2.1  Large-section histology image of an early carcinoma of the rectum.

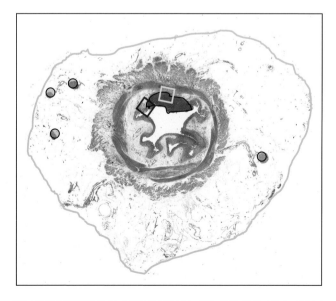

Fig. 2.1 d  Schematic guide to the morphologic details in the large section in Fig. 2.1.

## Case 2.2 Early Carcinoma of the Rectum

**Patient data:** 82-year-old man with rectal bleeding. Endoscopically, a 4 × 3-cm suspicious lesion was seen 13 cm from the anus. A preoperative diagnosis of invasive carcinoma was made on endoscopic biopsy.

**Surgical treatment:** Rectosigmoidal resection, no preoperative irradiation.

**Specimen:** 20-cm-long rectosigmoideum with a 4 × 3-cm exophytic tumor, 5 cm from the distal margin.

**Histopathologic diagnosis:** Moderately differentiated rectal adenocarcinoma infiltrating in but not beyond the lamina muscularis propria, 8 lymph nodes without signs of metastasis, radical excision, mesorectal margin 20 mm.

**TNM stage:** I (T2N0M0), Dukes A.

**Follow-up:** The patient died of heart failure 38 months after operation, without signs of recurrence of the tumor.

The exophytic tumor presented in Figure 2.**2** is an early invasive carcinoma infiltrating in but not through the lamina muscularis propria. The area of the tumor is colored red in the schematic image (Fig. 2.**2 d**). The level of infiltration in the muscularis propria is very well seen in the large histologic section. The deepest level of invasion is microscopically magnified in Figure 2.**2 a** (corresponding to the area of the yellow rectangle in Fig. 2.**2 d**). The level of infiltration – far beyond the lamina muscularis propria is easy to assess. Tumors operated at this early stage of development of rectal carcinoma have an excellent prognosis. Based on the abrupt transition of the normal epithelium into the tumor tissue, illustrated in Figure 2.**2 b** (corresponding to the area marked with the green arrow in Fig. 2.**2 d**), one may assume that the tumor, similar to the one discussed in the previous case, had developed without a stage of preexisting adenoma. These tumors, sometimes called „flat adenocarcinomas of the colorectum" may have a poorer prognosis than their „polypoid" counterparts, which develop through a precancerous stage of adenoma (Nasir et al. 2004).

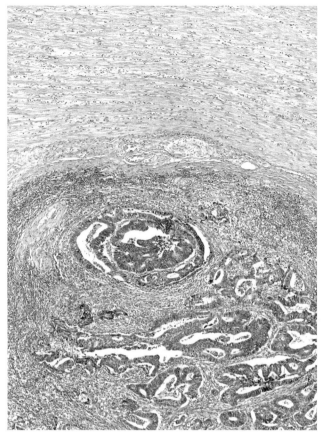

Fig. 2.**2 a**

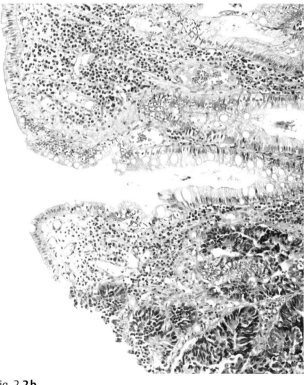

### Practical points

- Proper assessment of the level of invasion is essential for adequate staging of colorectal cancer.

Fig. 2.**2 b**

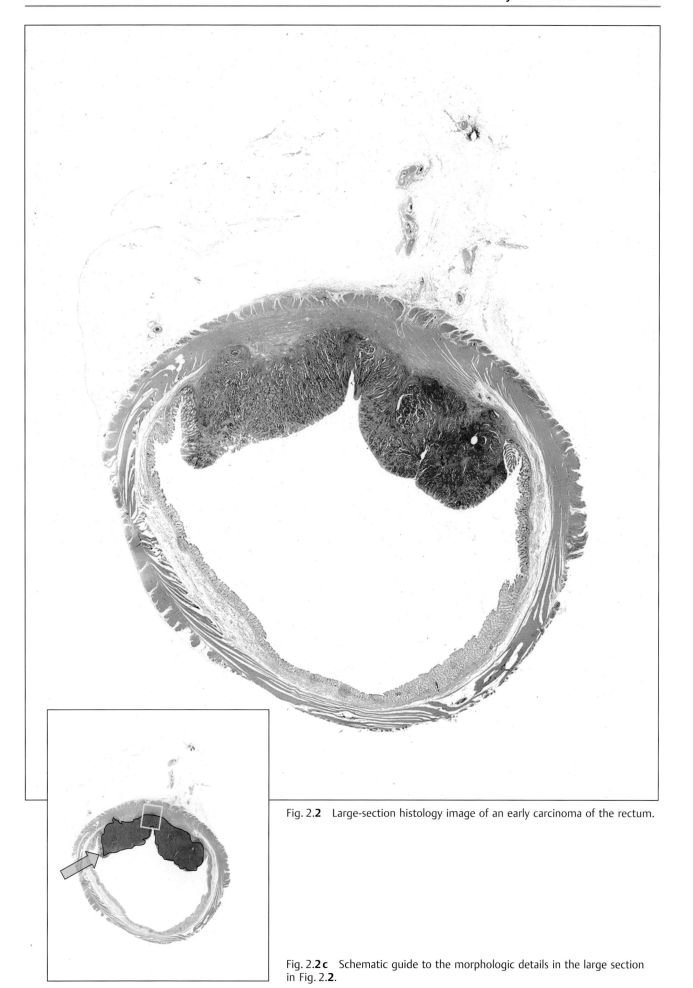

Fig. 2.**2**  Large-section histology image of an early carcinoma of the rectum.

Fig. 2.**2 c**  Schematic guide to the morphologic details in the large section in Fig. 2.**2**.

## Case 2.3 Early Colon Carcinoma, Dukes A

**Patient data:** 85-year-old man presenting with rectal bleeding. Endoscopically, a small polypoid lesion was found in the sigmoideum. A preoperative diagnosis of invasive carcinoma was made on endoscopic biopsy.

**Surgical treatment:** Sigmoideum resection, no preoperative irradiation.

**Specimen:** 11-cm-long sigmoideum with an exophytic tumor 20 mm in diameter, 4 cm from one of the margins.

**Histopathologic diagnosis:** Moderately differentiated adenocarcinoma infiltrating into but not beyond the lamina muscularis propria, 10 lymph nodes without signs of metastasis, radical excision.

**TNM stage:** I (T2N0M0), Dukes A.

**Follow-up:** 20 months, without signs of recurrence of colon carcinoma. The patient developed prostate cancer, diagnosed 10 months after surgery for colon cancer.

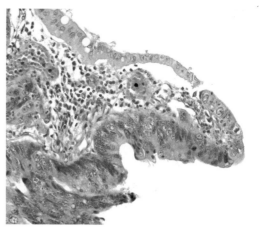

Fig. 2.**3a**

The large histologic section in Figure 2.**3** reliably demonstrates the level of invasion of the colon carcinoma (the tumor corresponds to the red-colored area in the schematic image, Fig. 2.**3c**), not reaching the outer layer of the lamina muscularis propria. The zone of transition between normal and neoplastic epithelium is illustrated in Figure 2.**3a** (microscopy image of the detail marked with the blue arrow in Fig. 2.**3c**). The deepest level of invasion corresponds to the area of the yellow rectangle in Figure 2.**3c** (microscopically magnified in Fig. 2.**3b**). The large section also included 5 lymph nodes free of metastasis (marked with green circles in Fig. 2.**3c**). The yellow arrow in Figure 2.**3c** indicates the mesenterial artery, the „root" of the surgical specimen.

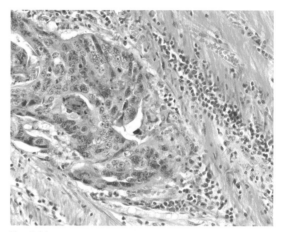

Fig. 2.**3b**

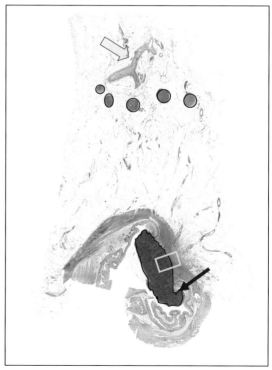

### Practical points

- Including structures of the mesenterium in addition to those of the bowel wall and the tumor may further assist in proper staging of the disease.

Fig. 2.**3c** Schematic guide to the morphologic details in the large section in Fig. 2.**3**.

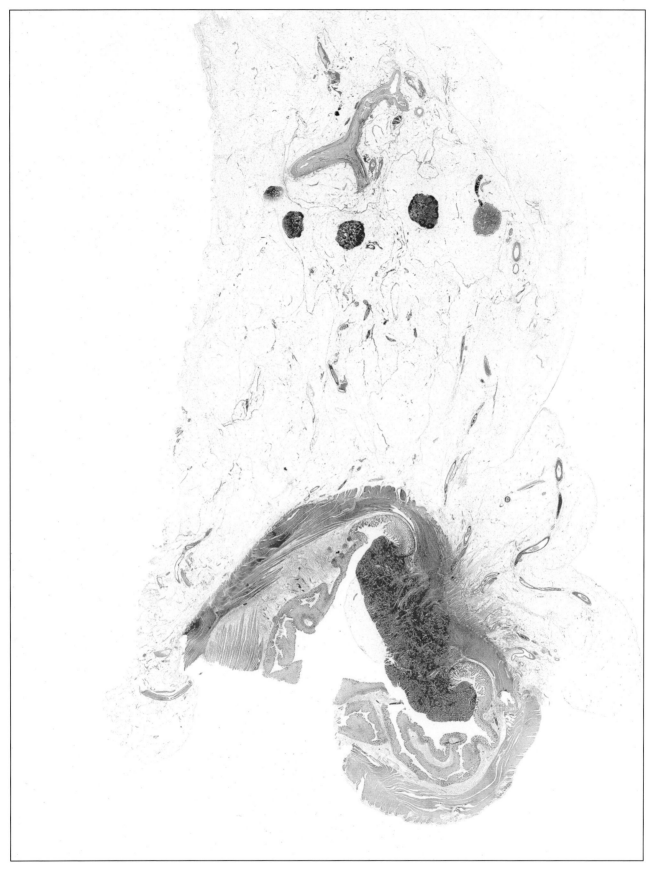

Fig. 2.**3**   Large-section histology image of an early colon carcinoma.

## Case 2.4 Early Rectal Carcinoma, Dukes A

**Patient data:** 70-year-old man presenting with rectal bleeding. Endoscopically, a small polypoid lesion was found in the rectum, 10 cm from the anus. A preoperative diagnosis of invasive carcinoma was made on endoscopic biopsy.

**Surgical treatment:** mesorectal resection, no preoperative irradiation.

**Specimen:** 18-cm-long rectum with an exophytic tumor 30 mm in diameter, 5 cm from the distal margin.

**Histopathologic diagnosis:** Moderately differentiated adenocarcinoma infiltrating into but not beyond the lamina muscularis propria, 12 lymph nodes without signs of metastasis, radical excision.

**TNM stage:** I (T2N0M0), Dukes A.

**Follow-up:** 54 months, no signs of disease recurrence.

This rectal carcinoma had obviously developed in an adenoma and infiltrated through the inner layer of the lamina muscularis propria into the outer layer, without reaching the perirectal tissue (Fig. 2.**4**). The tumor is marked with the red-colored area in the schematic image (Fig. 2.**4a**). Note the negative lymph node marked with green circle in Figure 2.**4a**. The specimen also included branches of the mesenteric artery (marked with yellow arrows in Fig. 2.**4a**). The circumferential margin, corresponding to the green-colored periphery of the schematic image, is well seen in the large histologic section and can be easily analyzed in all directions: at the lower edge, corresponding to the peritonealized ventral surface of the rectum, as well as at the upper part, corresponding to the surgical mesorectal margin.

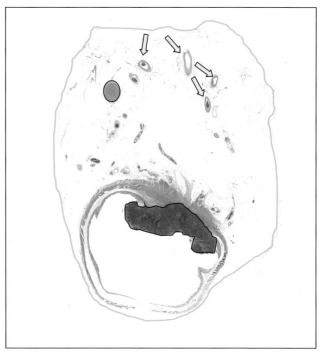

Fig. 2.**4a** Schematic guide to the morphologic details in the large section in Fig. 2.**4**.

### Practical points

- By including the continuous circumferential margin in one plane, the large histologic section is an ideal tool for assessing the radicality of mesorectal resection.

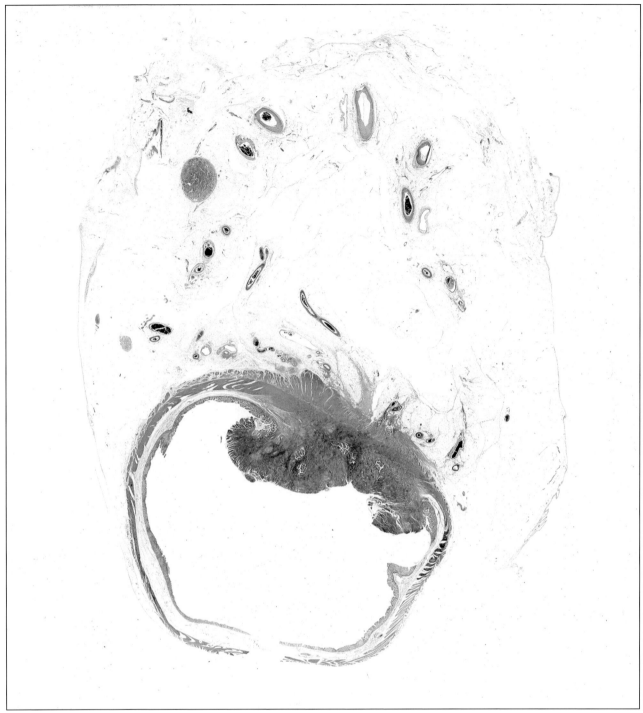

Fig. 2.**4**   Large-section histology image of an early rectal carcinoma.

## Case 2.5 Early Rectal Cancer

**Patient data:** 85-year-old man presenting with rectal bleeding. Endoscopically, a small polypoid lesion was found in the rectum, 7 cm from the anus. A preoperative diagnosis of invasive carcinoma was made on endoscopic biopsy.

**Surgical treatment:** Rectosigmoidal resection, no preoperative irradiation.

**Specimen:** 20-cm-long rectosigmoideum with a 5 × 3-cm ulcerated tumor, 2 cm from the distal margin.

**Histopathologic diagnosis:** Moderately differentiated adenocarcinoma infiltrating into but not beyond the lamina muscularis propria, 16 lymph nodes without signs of metastasis, radical excision.

**TNM stage:** I (T2N0M0), Dukes A.

**Follow-up:** 8 months, no signs of disease recurrence.

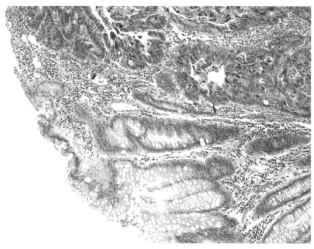

Fig. 2.**5a**

This large histologic section (Fig. 2.**5**) demonstrates an early carcinoma in the rectum infiltrating the lamina muscularis propria up to the border between the inner and outer muscle layers. The tumor destroyed about one half of the circumference of the mucosal surface. Note the lymph node in the mesorectum and the well-represented circumferential resection margin. The area of transition between the normal mucosa and the periphery of the tumor is magnified in Figure 2.**5a** (corresponding to the yellow-colored rectangle in the schematic image, Fig. 2.**5d**). Figure 2.**5b** represents a further detail of the invasive cancer in the same area. The deepest level of invasion was found in the area of the red rectangle in Figure 2.**5d** (microscopically magnified in Fig. 2.**5c**). The green arrow in Figure 2.**5d** marks the distance between the deepest level of invasion and the surgical margin (orange-colored in Fig. 2.**5d**), corresponding to the mesorectal resection margin. A free mesorectal resection margin has been found to be of crucial importance for proper surgical management of rectal cancers and for lowering the frequency of local recurrences. Thus, proper assessment of the distance indicated with the green arrow in Figure 2.**5d** is one of the most important tasks in modern surgical pathology.

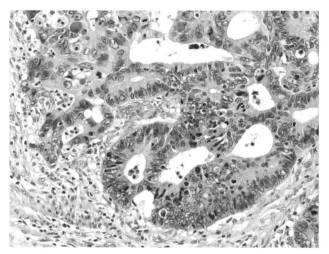

Fig. 2.**5b**

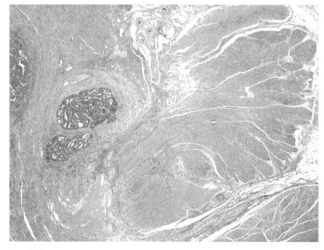

Fig. 2.**5c**

### Practical points

- One of the major advantages of the large section technique is inclusion of the circumferential margin of mesorectal resection specimens in one representative plane.

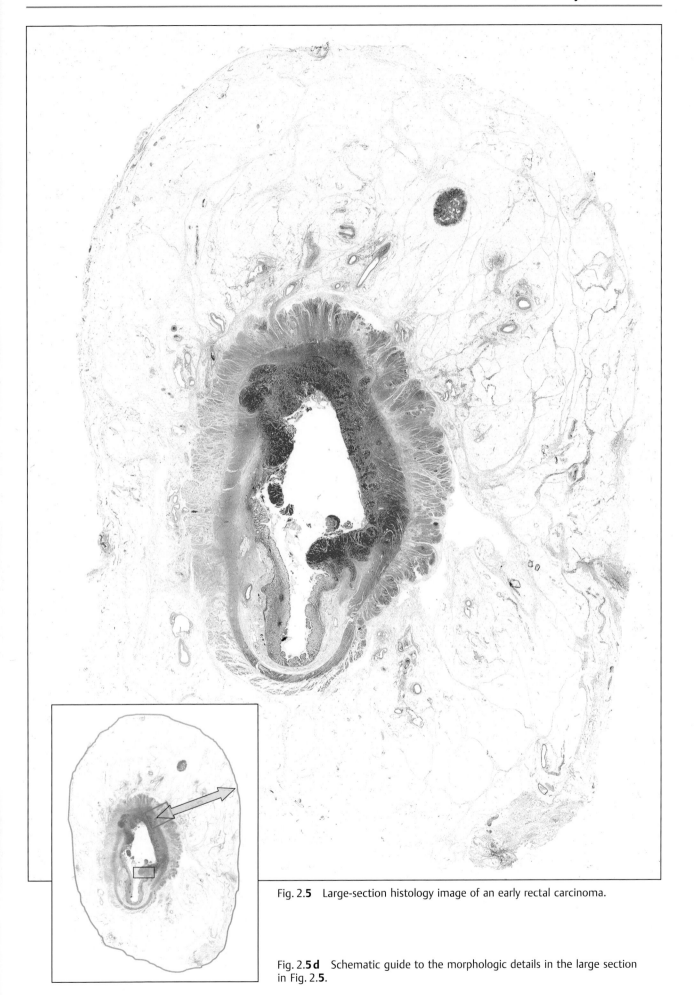

Fig. 2.5   Large-section histology image of an early rectal carcinoma.

Fig. 2.5 d   Schematic guide to the morphologic details in the large section in Fig. 2.5.

## Case 2.6 Early Rectal Cancer After Partial Endoscopic Resection

**Patient data:** 54-year-old man who underwent repeated endoscopic resection for a large rectal lesion diagnosed preoperatively as adenoma. The resected specimen contained a focus of an early invasive carcinoma, indicating the need for more radical surgical intervention.

**Surgical treatment:** Mesorectal resection, no preoperative irradiation.

**Specimen:** 21-cm-long rectum with a 2 × 2-cm irregular exophytic tumor, 2 cm from the distal margin.

**Histopathologic diagnosis:** Moderately differentiated adenocarcinoma infiltrating only the submucosa, previously partially resected endoscopically, 19 lymph nodes without signs of metastasis, radical excision.

**TNM stage:** I (T1N0M0), Dukes A.

**Follow-up:** 2 months, no signs of disease recurrence.

The large histologic section in Figure 2.**6** demonstrates an early rectal carcinoma, which has been previously partially resected endoscopically. The area of the previous resection is well seen in Figure 2.**6a**, showing ulcerated granulation tissue between the tumor (right lower edge of the image) and the regenerating mucosa (left lower edge of the image). The muscle layer is interrupted by fibrosis and scar formation. This image is a microscopic magnification of the area of the yellow rectangle in Figure 2.**6d**. The granulation tissue is further magnified in Figure 2.**6b**. A detail of the regenerating mucosa, corresponding to the green circle in the schematic image (Fig. 2.**6d**), is seen in Figure 2.**6c**. The specimen contained several small lymph nodes free of metastasis, which are marked with orange arrows in Figure2.**6d**.

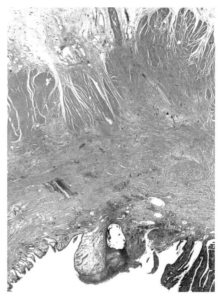

Fig. 2.**6a**

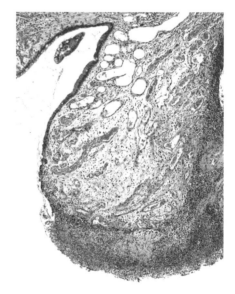

Fig. 2.**6b**

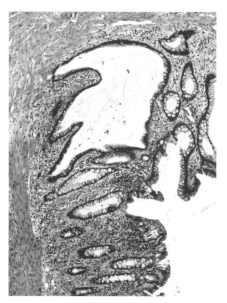

Fig. 2.**6c**

### Practical points

- In this particular case, the large section reliably demonstrates the effects of the previous endoscopic resection, as well as the rests of the tumor.
- Regenerative changes and scarring are regularly seen after endoscopic resection of intestinal lesions.

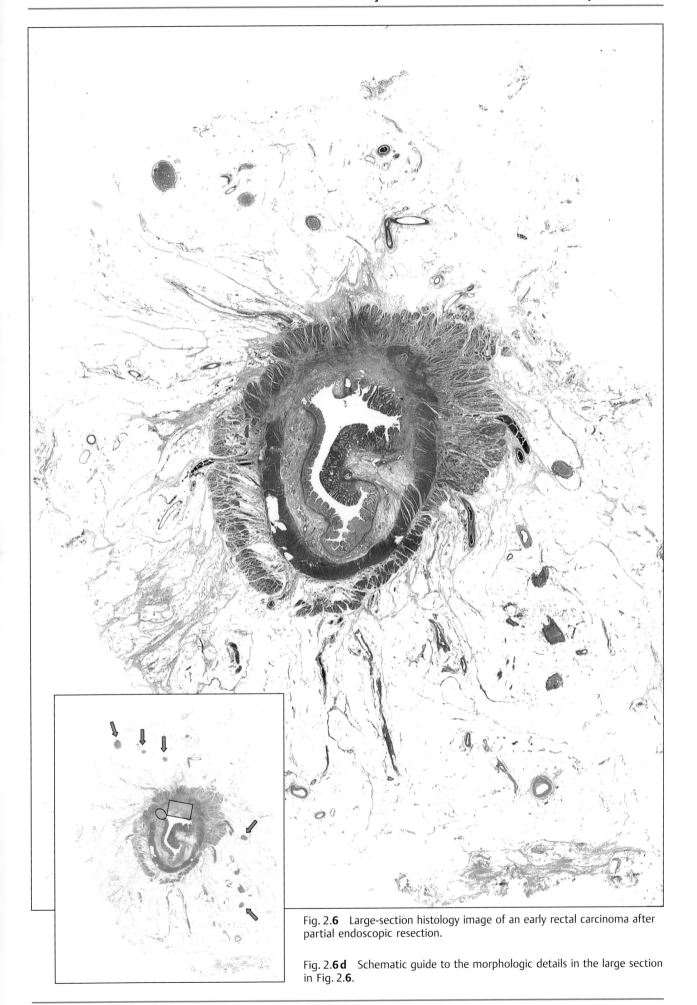

**Fig. 2.6** Large-section histology image of an early rectal carcinoma after partial endoscopic resection.

**Fig. 2.6d** Schematic guide to the morphologic details in the large section in Fig. 2.**6**.

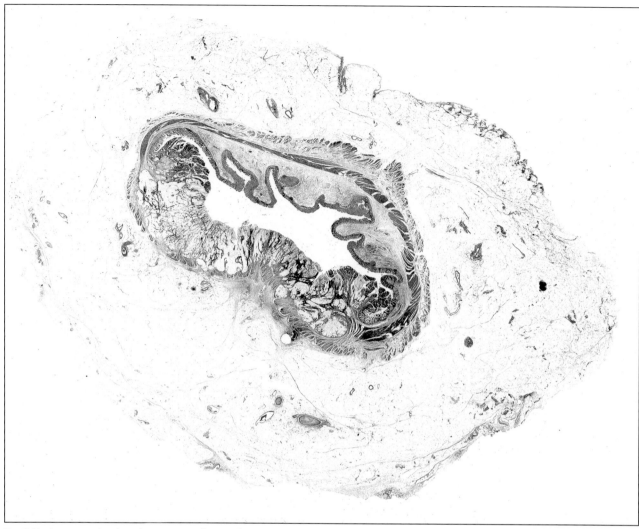

Fig. 2.**7**  Large-section histology image of an early mucinous rectal carcinoma, Dukes A.

## Cases 2.7 and 2.8 Comparison of the Level of Invasion in Two Different Cases of Mucinous Carcinoma

The large histologic section in Figure 2.**7** demonstrates a mucinous carcinoma infiltrating the muscular layer of the rectum but respecting the outer border of the lamina muscularis propria. The tumor is classified as Dukes A according to the Dukes system and T2 according to the TNM classification.

The other case of mucinous carcinoma of the rectum, shown in the large section in Figure 2.**8**, is a tumor that did not infiltrate beyond the level of the lamina muscularis propria, but reached the border between the muscular layer and the pericolic tissue. This is a borderline case between Dukes A or B (T2 or T3). In cases like this one, or if the infiltration is massive, examination of the specimen at different levels and serial sectioning of the paraffin-embedded slices are recommended for proper staging.

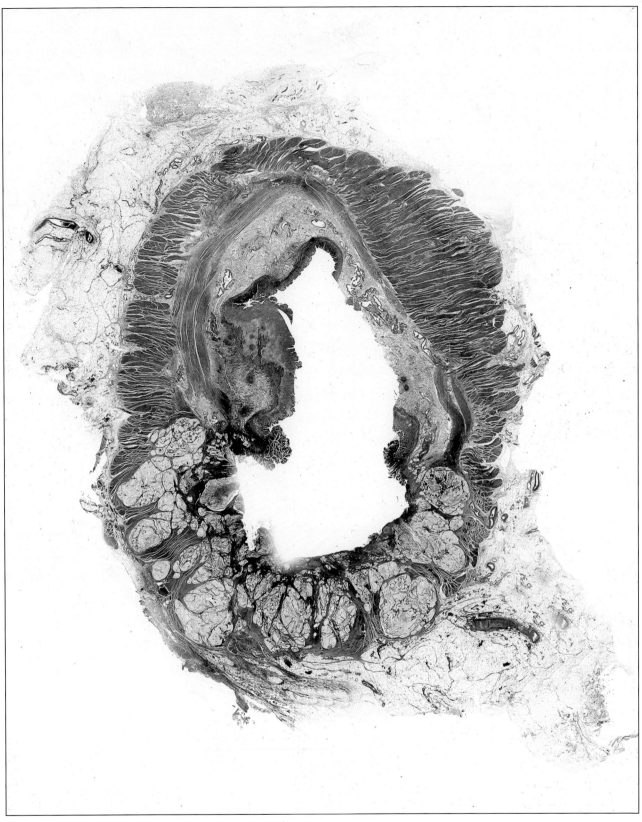

Fig. 2.**8**   Large-section histology image of a mucinous colon carcinoma.

## Case 2.9 „Early" Rectal Carcinoma with Vascular Invasion

**Patient data:** 71-year-old woman with diffuse abdominal pain. A small tumor was found endoscopically in her rectum, 10 cm from the anus. The diagnosis of invasive carcinoma was made on endoscopic biopsy.

**Surgical treatment:** Rectosigmoidal resection, no preoperative irradiation.

**Specimen:** 30-cm-long rectosigmoideum with a 2× 1-cm exophytic tumor, 3 cm from the distal margin.

**Histopathologic diagnosis:** Moderately differentiated adenocarcinoma infiltrating only the submucosa and the inner part of the lamina muscularis propria. Vascular invasion, 9 lymph nodes without signs of metastasis, radical excision.

**TNM stage:** I (T2N0M0V1), Dukes A.

**Follow-up:** 24 months, no signs of recurrence of the rectal carcinoma. The patient developed breast carcinoma 13 months after diagnosis of the rectal cancer.

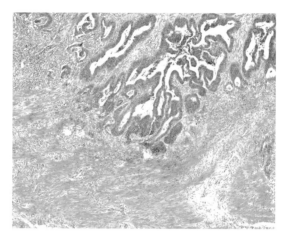

Fig. 2.**9a**

The carcinoma of the rectum presented in Figure 2.**9** (corresponding to the red-colored area in the schematic image, Fig. 2.**9d**) invaded only the inner layer of the muscularis propria and seemed to be an early rectal cancer on macroscopic examination. The assumed deepest level of invasion is histologically magnified in Figure 2.**9a**. However, in the central part of the lesion, a few tumor structures disrupted the outer layer of the muscle coat and found their way to a vascular space. The corresponding structures are located in the area of the blue ellipse in Figure 2.**9d** and are histologically magnified in Figure 2.**9b, c**. The TNM classification uses the category of V1 for vascular invasion seen only on microscopy. These tumors, although categorized as Dukes A and TNM stage I, may have a poor prognosis. The mesorectal resection margin is well demonstrated in the large histologic section in Figure 2.**9** and is free of cancer. The yellow arrow in the schematic image marks a small lymph node.

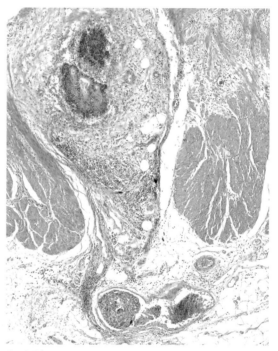

Fig. 2.**9b**

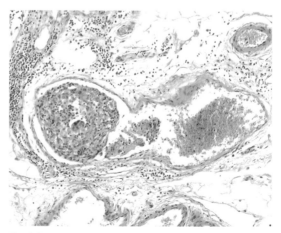

### Practical points

- Inclusion of a large area of the mesorectal/mesocolic tissue is a further advantage of the large sections, as vascular invasion can be easily seen.

Fig. 2.**9c**

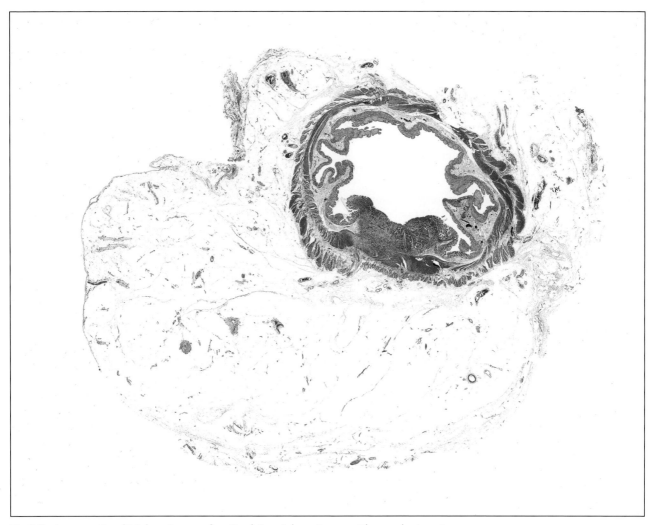

Fig. 2.**9** Large-section histology image of an "early" rectal carcinoma with vascular invasion.

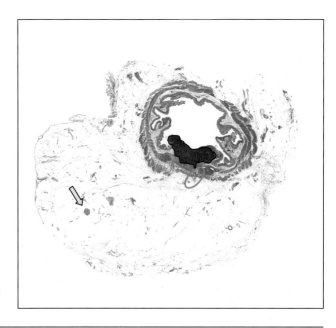

Fig. 2.**9 d** Schematic guide to the morphologic details in the large section in Fig. 2.**9**.

# Case 2.10 „Early" Rectal Carcinoma with Metastasis

**Patient data:** 71-year-old woman with rectal bleeding. Endoscopically, a small ulcerated lesion was found in her rectum, 11 cm from the anus. A preoperative diagnosis of invasive carcinoma was made on endoscopic biopsy.

**Surgical treatment:** Preoperative irradiation and rectosigmoidal resection.

**Specimen:** 21-cm-long rectosigmoideum with an ulcerated tumor 15 mm in diameter and 5 cm from the distal margin.

**Histopathologic diagnosis:** Moderately differentiated rectal adenocarcinoma infiltrating into but not beyond the lamina muscularis propria. Three of the 10 examined lymph nodes contained metastases. Radical excision.

**TNM stage:** IIIA (T2N1M0), Dukes AC.

**Follow-up:** 24 months with an episode of rectal bleeding due to biopsy verified solitary rectal ulcer. No signs of recurrence of the cancer.

The small invasive carcinoma of the rectum, shown in Figure 2.**10** (corresponding to the red-colored area in Fig. 2.**10c**), invaded only the submucosa and the inner layer of the lamina muscularis propria. The deepest level of invasion (area of the yellow rectangle in Fig. 2.**10c**) is microscopically magnified in Figure 2.**10a**. The tumor was deeply ulcerated. Although preoperative irradiation often diminishes the size of a tumor and may lead to histologic down-staging of the disease, in this particular case the intact outer layer of lamina muscularis propria indicates that the level of invasion is properly documented and was always restricted to the muscular layer. The early stage of development of the invasive tumor contrasts with the unexpected presence of lymph node metastases. One of the metastatic nodes (marked with the green circle in Fig. 2.**10c** and magnified in Fig. 2.**10b**) is present in the large section (Fig. 2.**10**). A minority of superficially infiltrating colorectal carcinomas exhibits metastatic capacity. These tumors are sometimes designated as „Dukes AC" cancers.

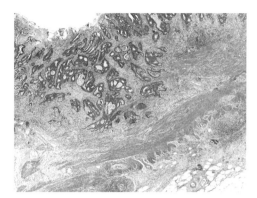

Fig. 2.**10a**

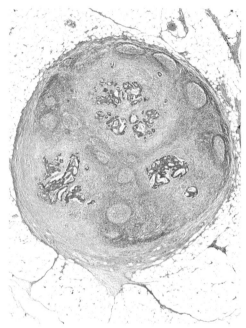

Fig. 2.**10b**

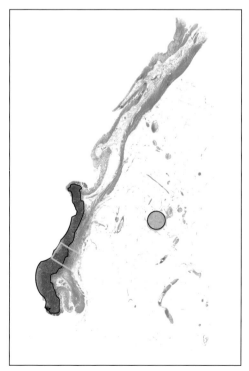

Fig. 2.**10c** Schematic guide to the morphologic details in the large section in Fig. 2.**10**.

## Practical points

- By showing the deepest level of invasion together with a number of perirectal lymph nodes, the large section offers a contiguous image for diagnosing and staging primary colorectal carcinomas.

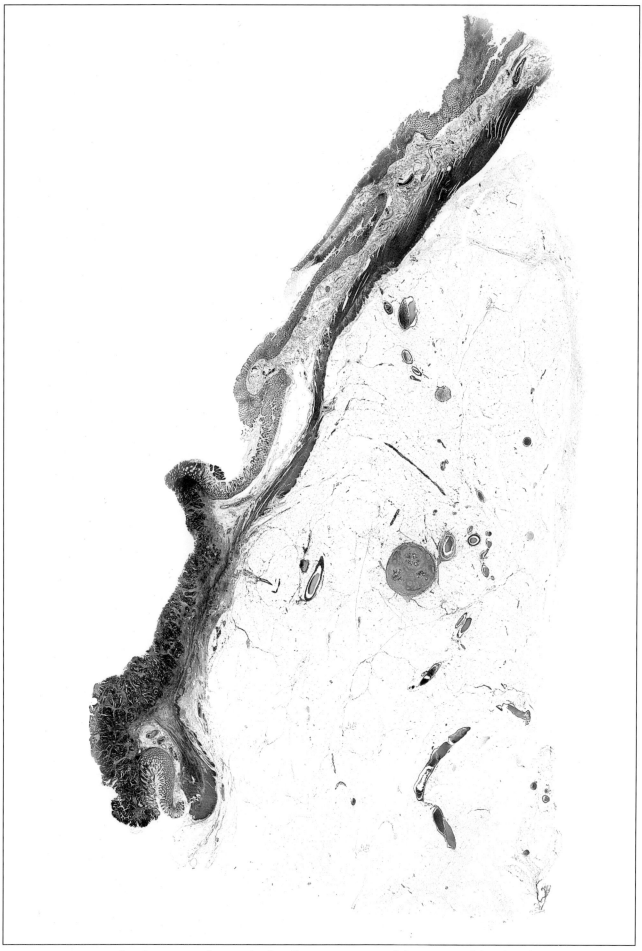

Fig. 2.**10**   Large-section histology image of a superficially infiltrating carcinoma of the rectum with lymph node metastasis.

## Case 2.11 Rectal Carcinoma, Dukes B

**Patient data:** 59-year-old woman with rectal bleeding. A small tumor was found endoscopically in her rectum, 7 cm from the anus. The diagnosis of invasive carcinoma was made on endoscopic biopsy.
**Surgical treatment:** Mesorectal resection, no preoperative irradiation.
**Specimen:** 18-cm-long rectum with a 3 × 2-cm exophytic tumor, 1 cm from the distal margin.
**Histopathologic diagnosis:** Moderately differentiated adenocarcinoma infiltrating through the lamina muscularis propria, 12 lymph nodes without signs of metastasis, radical excision.
**TNM stage:** IIA (T3N0M0), Dukes B.
**Follow-up:** 12 months, no signs of disease recurrence.

The large histologic section shown in Figure 2.**11** demonstrates a carcinoma (corresponding to the red-colored surface in the schematic image, Fig. 2.**11 d**) that infiltrated through the muscular wall of the rectum only in a very limited area. The abrupt transition from normal to neoplastic epithelium is illustrated in Figure 2.**11 a**, which is a microscopic magnification of the area marked with the yellow arrow in Figure 2.**11 d**. The deepest level of infiltration is seen in the area indicated by the blue rectangle in Figure 2.**11 d** (magnified in Fig. 2.**11 b**). The tumor infiltrated using the perivascular tissue of a larger blood vessel. The area of the vasculature penetrating the muscle coat of the intestine represents a point of low resistance where transmural infiltration may start. Figure 2.**11 c** is a high-power magnification of the adenocarcinoma.

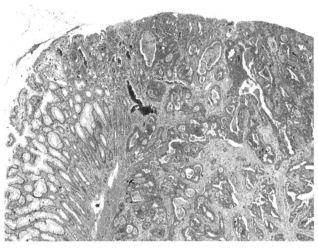

Fig. 2.**11 a**

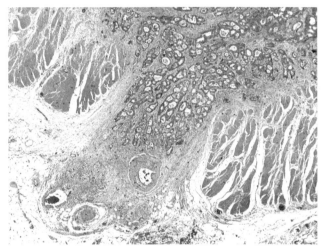

Fig. 2.**11 b**

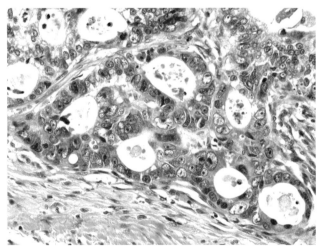

Fig. 2.**11 c**

### Practical points

- The large histologic section demonstrates not only the level of invasion, but also the pattern of invasive tumor growth.
- The area of the vasculature penetrating the muscle coat of the intestine represents a weak point where transmural infiltration may start.

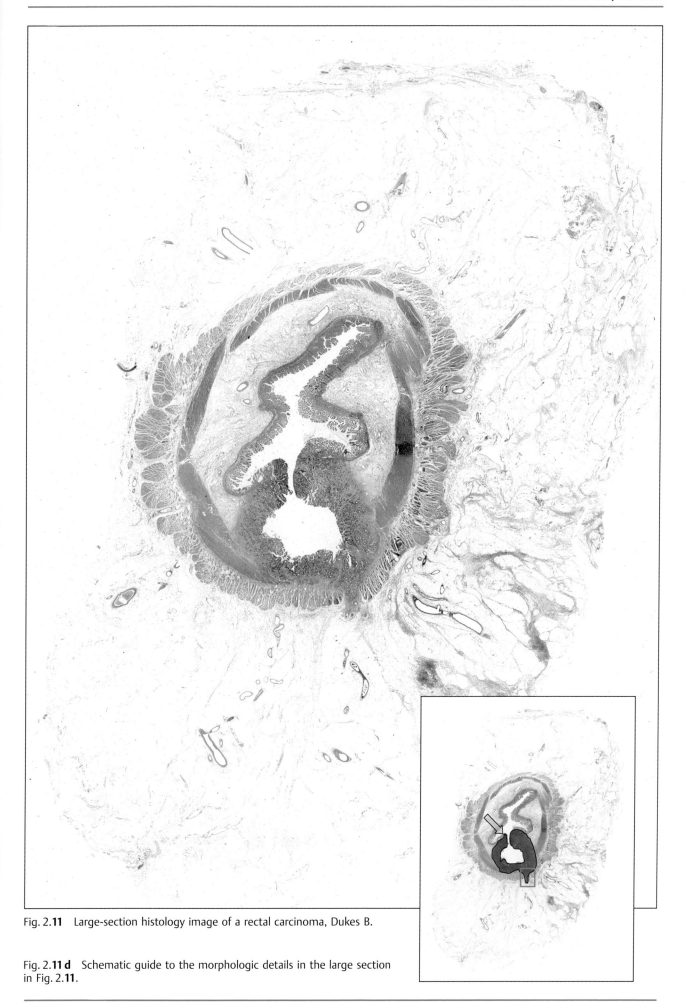

Fig. 2.11  Large-section histology image of a rectal carcinoma, Dukes B.

Fig. 2.11 d  Schematic guide to the morphologic details in the large section in Fig. 2.11.

## Case 2.12 Early Rectal Cancer: The Rectum Is Adherent to the Uterus

**Patient data:** 69-year-old woman with rectal bleeding. A small tumor was found endoscopically in her rectum, 10 cm from the anus. The diagnosis of invasive carcinoma was made on endoscopic biopsy.

**Surgical treatment:** Intraoperatively, the surgeon found that the anterior surface of the rectum was adherent to the uterine corpus. As direct overgrowth of the tumor was suspected, the rectum was resected together with the uterus and the uterine adnexa. No preoperative irradiation.

**Specimen:** 20-cm-long rectum with a 3 × 2-cm exophytic tumor, 4 cm from the distal margin. Adherent 6-cm-long uterus with adnexa.

**Histopathologic diagnosis:** Moderately differentiated adenocarcinoma of the rectum, infiltrating in but not extending beyond the lamina muscularis propria, 10 lymph nodes without signs of metastasis, radical excision. Peritoneal endometriosis.

**TNM stage:** I (T2N0M0), Dukes A.

**Follow-up:** 22 months, no signs of disease recurrence.

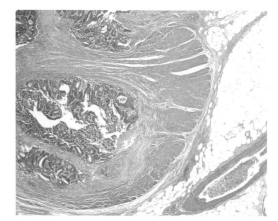

Fig. 2.**12 a**

This large histologic section (Fig. 2.**12**) is a transection of the uterine corpus and the rectum, which have adhered to each other. During surgery, the fibrous adhesions gave a false impression of continuous tumor spread from rectum to uterus, indicating the need for a more radical surgical intervention. The histologic work-up demonstrated a Dukes A adenocarcinoma in the rectum (corresponding to the yellow-colored area in the schematic image, Fig. 2.**12 e**), respecting the borders of the rectal wall. Figure 2.**12 a** is a microscopic magnification of the deepest level of invasion, demonstrating that the outer part of the muscularis propria is intact. Figure 2.**12 b** represents further magnification of the tumor tissue. The perirectal fatty tissue contained reactive lymph nodes (marked with red circles in Fig. 2.**12 e**). The peripheral border of the perirectal fatty tissue is marked green in Figure 2.**12 e** and the peripheral border of the uterine corpus red. The frontal surface of the rectum and the dorsal surface of the uterine corpus were connected to each other by strands of fibrous tissue (marked with the green rectangle in the schematic image). The same area contained mesothelial inclusion cysts (Fig. 2.**12 c**) and small islands of endometriosis (Fig. 2.**12 d**).

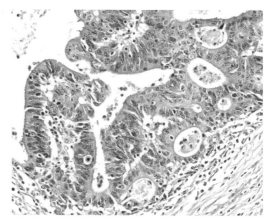

Fig. 2.**12 b**

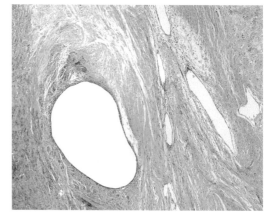

Fig. 2.**12 c**

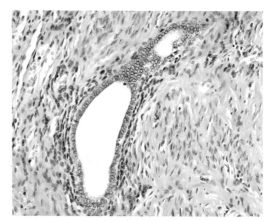

Fig. 2.**12 d**

### Practical points

- A large histologic section may include a transection of several organs, allowing direct assessment of the presence or absence of continuous tumor spread („contact metastasis").

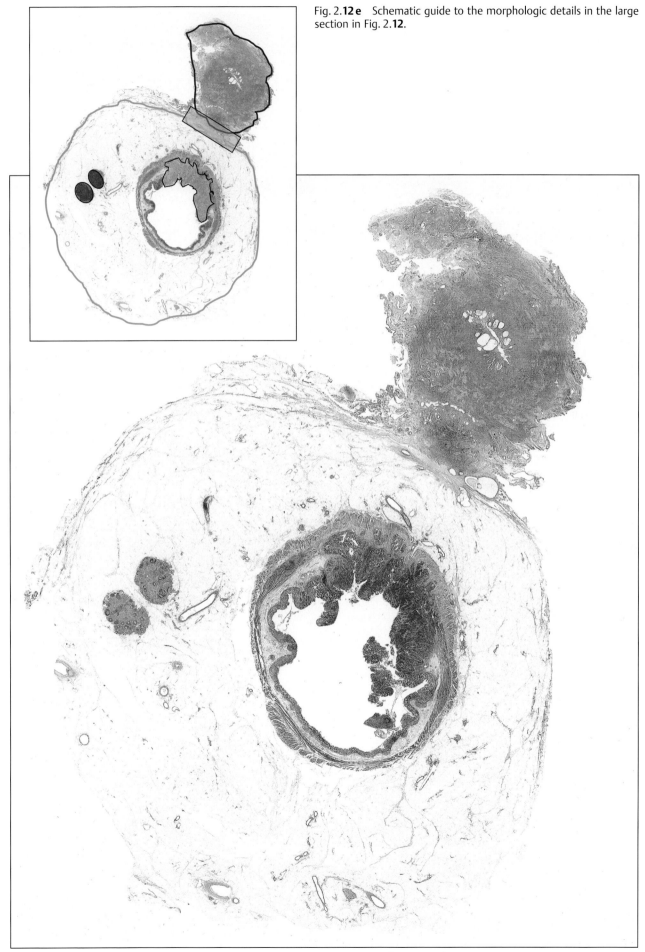

Fig. 2.**12 e**   Schematic guide to the morphologic details in the large section in Fig. 2.**12**.

Fig. 2.**12**   Large-section histology image of a rectal carcinoma: the rectum is adherent to the uterine corpus.

## Case 2.13 Colon Carcinoma with Intratumoral Heterogeneity

**Patient data:** **70**-year-old-man presenting with anemia. Endoscopic examination revealed a small polypoid tumor in the cecum, diagnosed preoperatively as adenoma with severe dysplasia. During laparotomy, multiple peritoneal metastases were seen.

**Surgical treatment:** Right hemicolectomy, resection of the omentum, no preoperative irradiation.

**Specimen:** 35-cm-long segment of the colon with a part of the terminal ileum, containing a 4-cm exophytic tumor in the cecum.

**Histopathologic diagnosis:** Moderately differentiated colon adenocarcinoma infiltrating through the lamina muscularis propria. Multiple metastases in 5 of 11 examined lymph nodes and in the omentum.

**TNM stage:** IV (T4N2M1).

**Follow-up:** 3 months, no signs of disease recurrence.

The large histologic section in Figure 2.**13** shows a carcinoma of the cecum with obvious intratumoral heterogeneity. This is illustrated by the two different colors indicating the area of the tumor in the schematic image (Fig. 2.**13 f**). The red-colored area corresponds to the part of the tumor exhibiting structures of a usual adenocarcinoma of intestinal type developing in an adenoma. This part of the tumor is also seen in Figure 2.**13 a**, which is a microscopic magnification of the area of the green rectangle in Figure 2.**13 f**. The other part of the same tumor (corresponding to the yellow-colored area in Fig. 2.**13 f**) is histologically different and represents a papillary adenocarcinoma with numerous psammoma-body-type microcalcifications. The interface of the two different histologic appearances of the same tumor is seen in Figure 2.**13 b** (corresponding to the area of the white rectangle in Fig. 2.**13 f**). The papillary part of the tumor is microscopically magnified in Figure 2.**13 c**. Immunohistohemical reactions on cytokeratin 20 (Fig. 2.**13 d**) and cytokeratin 7 (Fig. 2.**13 e**) further demonstrate the differences in the phenotype of the two tumor-cell populations within the same tumor (Tot 2002). The case was included here to illustrate a rare problem in classification of colorectal tumors with intratumoral heterogeneity. A collision tumor representing a metastasis of a papillary carcinoma into a Dukes A colorectal cancer was the other differential diagnostic option. Papillary carcinomas with psammoma bodies are a rarity in the colon (Nakayama et al 1997), but are very frequent in the ovaries, thyroid gland and peritoneum. Meticulous clinical and radiological investigations carried out in the present case ruled out the presence of another primary carcinoma. Thus, the tumor was classified as advanced colon carcinoma with obvious intratumoral heterogeneity.

### Practical points

● In this particular case, the large section included two different tumor-cell populations within the same tumor and reliably demonstrated the intratumoral heterogeneity, which allowed proper classification of the tumor.

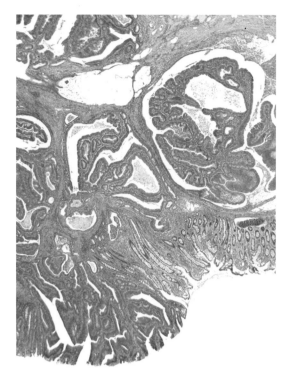

Fig. 2.**13 a**

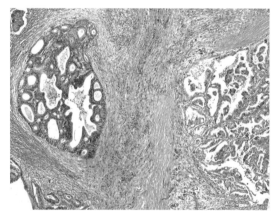

Fig. 2.**13 b**

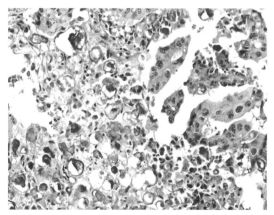

Fig. 2.**13 c**

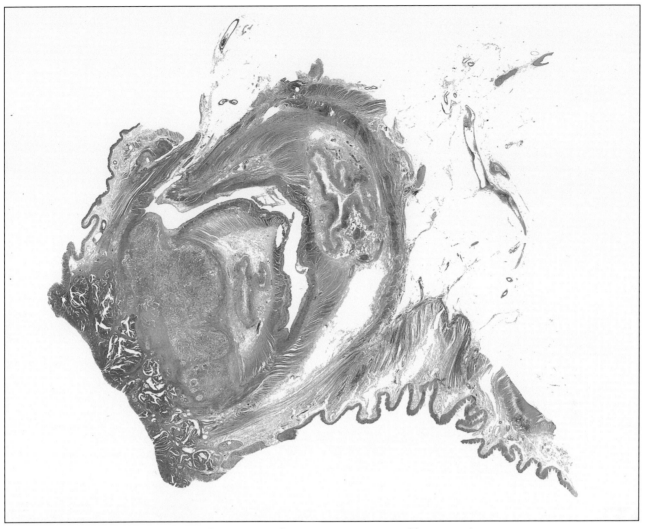

Fig. 2.**13**   Large-section histology image of a carcinoma demonstrating intratumoral heterogeneity.

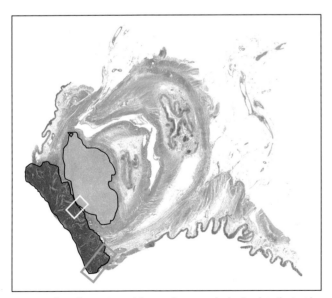

Fig. 2.**13 f**   Schematic guide to the morphologic details in the large section in Fig. 2.**13**.

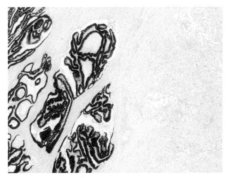

Fig. 2.**13 d**

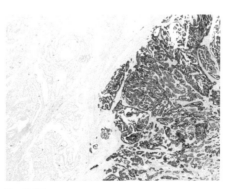

Fig. 2.**13 e**

# 3 Advanced Colorectal Cancer

## Case 3.1 Infiltrating Colon Carcinoma, Dukes B

**Patient data:** 77-year-old male patient presenting with sideropenic anemia. An ulcerated tumor was found endoscopically in the cecum, diagnosed as invasive carcinoma on preoperative biopsy.

**Surgical treatment:** Right hemicolectomy, no preoperative irradiation.

**Specimen:** 36-cm-long colon segment with a 5-cm part of the terminal ileum containing an exophytic tumor in the cecum 4 cm in diameter.

**Histopathologic diagnosis:** Moderately differentiated adenocarcinoma infiltrating through the lamina muscularis propria into the pericolic tissue, 13 lymph nodes without signs of metastasis, radical excision.

**TNM stage:** IIA (T3N0M0), Dukes B.

**Follow-up:** 49 months, no signs of disease recurrence.

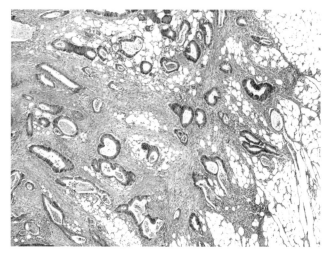

Fig. 3.**1a**

Infiltration of the tumor structures beyond the level of the muscularis propria into the subserosa or into the pericolic/perirectal tissue (as illustrated in Fig. 3.**1a**) indicates B stage in Dukes' classification. Many other classification systems, including the TNM classification, recognize this level of infiltration as a crucial unfavorable prognostic factor. As was already demonstrated, a large histologic section, taken in the plane of the deepest infiltration of the tumor, shows the level of infiltration without the aid of a microscope. The large section shown in Figure 3.**1** demonstrates an infiltrating carcinoma of the cecum, corresponding to the red-colored area in the schematic image (Fig. 3.**1b**). The deepest tumor structures infiltrating into the fatty tissue are microscopically magnified in Figure 3.**1a**. Note the reactive lymph nodes (indicated with green arrows in Fig. 3.**1b**). Since the tumor developed in the cecum, a transection of the terminal part of the ileum (indicated with the yellow arrow in Fig. 3.**1b**) was also included in the large section.

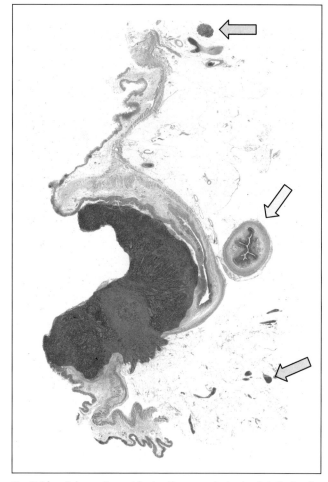

Fig. 3.**1b** Schematic guide to the morphologic details in the large section in Fig. 3.**1**.

### Practical points

- Taken in the plane of the deepest invasion, the large histologic section reliably demonstrates the level of primary tumor growth.
- Inclusion of a large area of the pericolic/perirectal tissue is a further advantage of large histologic sections, which allow the pattern and extent of the invasion to be easily assessed.

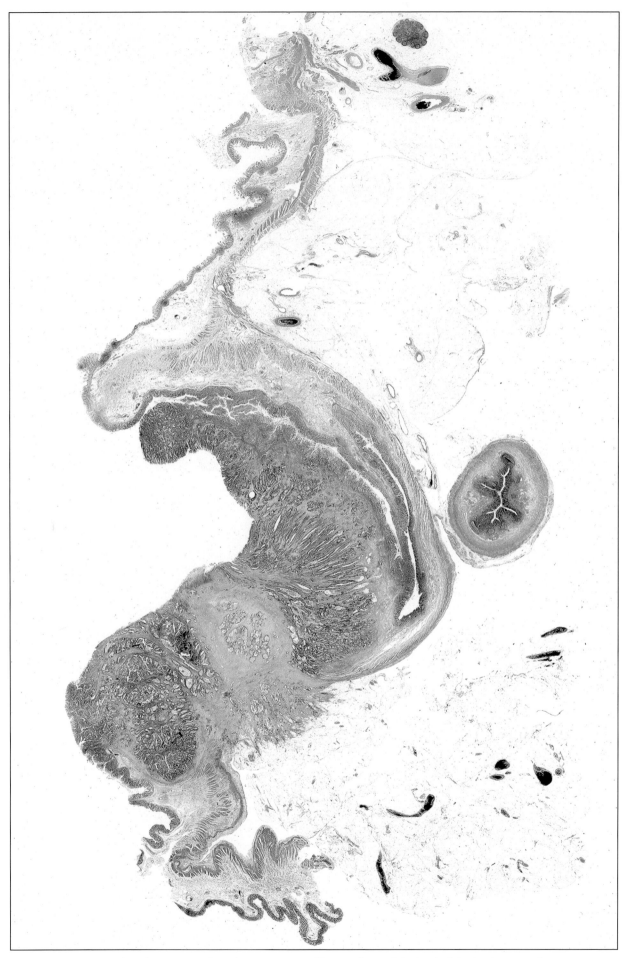

Fig. 3.**1** Large-section histology image of a colon carcinoma infiltrating beyond the level of the lamina muscularis propria.

## Case 3.2 Rectal Carcinoma That Developed in a Villous Adenoma

**Patient data:** 72-year-old female patient presenting with rectal bleeding. An ulcerated tumor was found endoscopically in her rectum 7 cm from the anus, diagnosed as invasive carcinoma on endoscopic biopsy.

**Surgical treatment:** Mesorectal resection, no preoperative irradiation.

**Specimen:** 18-cm-long rectum with a 6 × 5-cm partly exophytic, partly ulcerated tumor, 2 cm from the distal margin.

**Histopathologic diagnosis:** Moderately differentiated adenocarcinoma infiltrating through the lamina muscularis propria into the pericolic tissue. Ten lymph nodes without signs of metastasis. Radical excision.

**TNM stage:** IIA (T3N0M0), Dukes B.

**Follow-up:** 17 months, no signs of disease recurrence.

In this particular case, the large histologic section (Fig. 3.**2**) demonstrates a villous adenoma covering the anterior part of the rectal circumference and an invasive carcinoma that developed in the adenoma covering the posterior half. The villous structures of the adenoma (corresponding to the area of the blue circle in Fig. 3.**2e**) are also seen magnified in Figure 3.**2a**. The interface of the structures of the adenoma and the carcinoma is microscopically magnified in Figure 3.**2b**, corresponding to the area of the red rectangle in the schematic image (Fig. 3.**2e**). The cancer infiltrated beyond the level of the lamina muscularis propria, interrupting the muscle layer at several points, two of which are magnified in Figure 3.**2c,d** (corresponding to the green and yellow rectangles in the schematic image, Fig. 3.**2e**, respectively). The blue arrow indicates the free mesorectal resection margin. A narrow white line in Figure 3.**2e** marks the border between the adenoma (under the line) and the carcinoma (above the line).

### Practical points

- The large histological sections facilitate the assessment of the mesorectal margin.
- The spatial and quantitative relation of the carcinoma to the pre-existent adenoma is also easy to demonstrate using this technique.

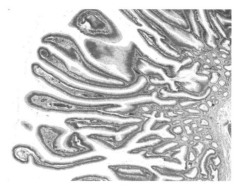

Fig. 3.**2a**

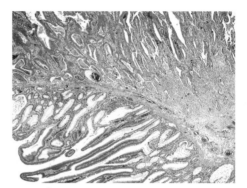

Fig. 3.**2b**

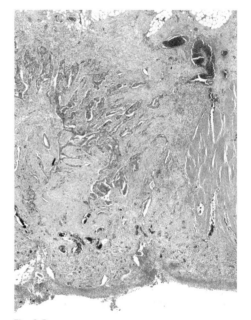

Fig. 3.**2c**

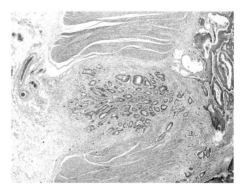

Fig. 3.**2d**

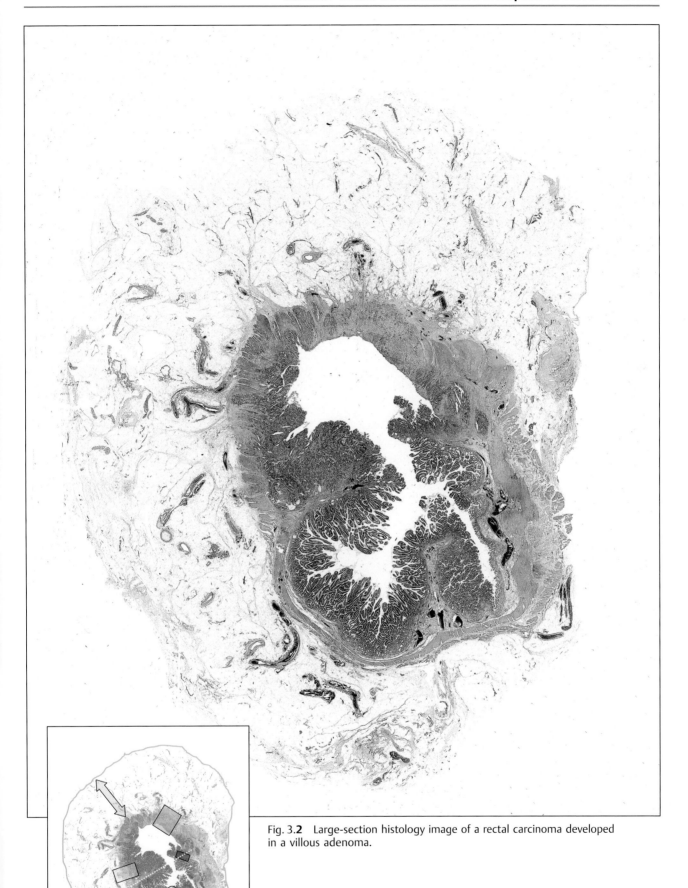

Fig. 3.**2**    Large-section histology image of a rectal carcinoma developed in a villous adenoma.

Fig. 3.**2e**    Schematic guide to the morphologic details in the large section in Fig. 3.**2**.

## Case 3.3 Rectal Carcinoma, Dukes C

**Patient data:** 77-year-old male presenting with watery diarrhea. A large tumor was found endoscopically in his rectum, 10 cm from the anus, diagnosed as invasive carcinoma on endoscopic biopsy.
**Surgical treatment:** Preoperative irradiation and mesorectal resection.
**Specimen:** 25-cm-long rectum with an 8 × 7-cm ulcerated tumor, 5 cm from the distal margin.
**Histopathologic diagnosis:** Moderately differentiated adenocarcinoma infiltrating through the lamina muscularis propria into the pericolic tissue. Three of the 14 examined lymph nodes contained metastasis. Radical excision.
**TNM stage:** IIIB (T3N1M0), Dukes C.
**Follow-up:** 46 months, no signs of disease recurrence.

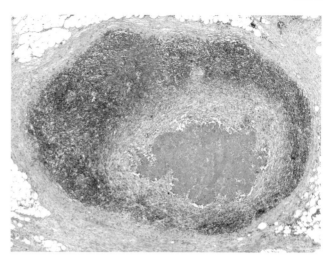

Fig. 3.**3a**

The large histologic section in Figure 3.**3** demonstrates an advanced rectal carcinoma (corresponding to the red-colored area in the schematic image, Fig. 3.**3b**), which had developed in a tubulovillous adenoma. The rests of the adenoma are well seen on the periphery of the tumor. The cancer infiltrated through the muscular wall following the perivascular spaces. Examination of the tumor after preoperative irradiation showed some regression of the cancer as well as peritumoral fibrosis. The two lymph nodes in the specimen (marked with the blue arrows in Fig. 3.**3b**) were free of metastases. However, the third lymph node (marked with the yellow rectangle) contained a necrotic mass corresponding to a necrotic metastasis after irradiation. This node is histologically magnified in Figure 3.**3a**.

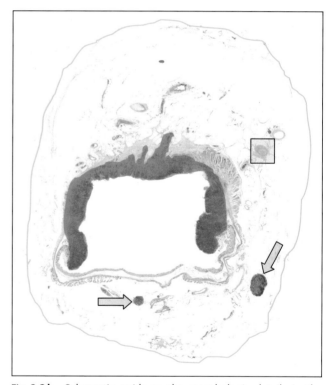

Fig. 3.**3b** Schematic guide to the morphologic details in the large section in Fig. 3.**3**.

### Practical points

- Taken in the plane of the deepest invasion, the large histologic section reliably demonstrates the level of primary tumor growth and allows the effects of irradiation to be assessed.

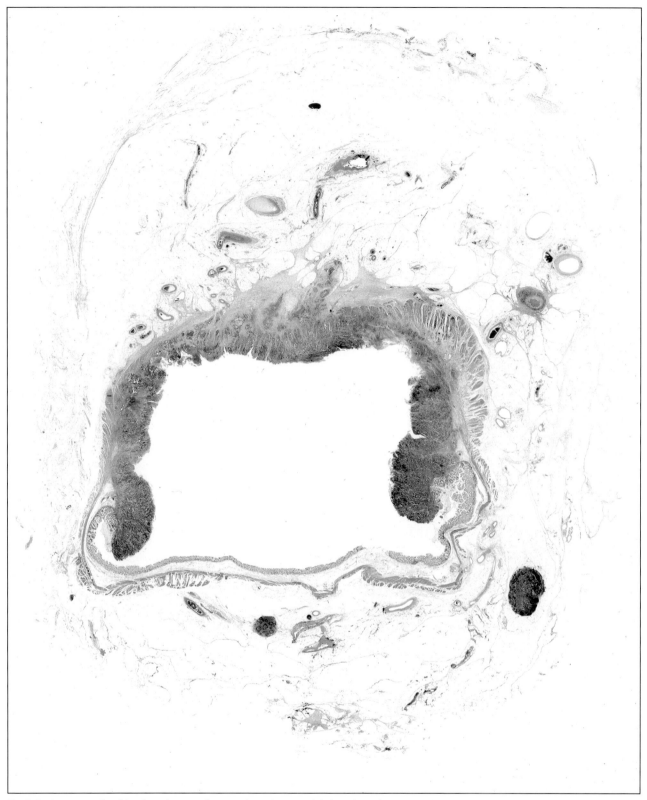

Fig. 3.**3**  Large-section histology image of a rectal carcinoma with lymph node metastasis.

## Case 3.4 Mucinous Carcinoma of the Colon

**Patient data:** 66-year-old man with sideropenic anemia and celiac disease. A large tumor was found endoscopically in the area of the ileocecal valve. The endoscopic biopsy contained only adenoma structures.

**Surgical treatment:** Ileocecal resection, no preoperative irradiation. Liver metastases were seen on laparotomy.

**Specimen:** 12-cm-long ileocecal specimen with a 6-cm-long appendix. The cecum contained an exophytic 7 × 5-cm tumor, 6 cm from the distal margin.

**Histopathologic diagnosis:** Well-differentiated mucinous adenocarcinoma infiltrating through the lamina muscularis propria into the pericolic tissue. Four of 10 lymph nodes with metastases. Radical excision.

**TNM stage:** IV (T3N2M1), Dukes C.

**Follow-up:** Died of the disease 9 months after the operation.

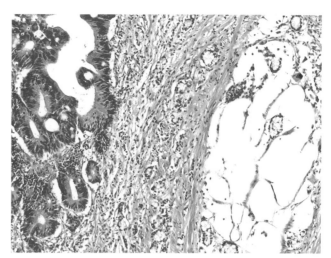

Fig. 3.**4a**

The mucinous carcinoma demonstrated in Figure 3.**4** had also developed in a villous adenoma. Both the structures of the adenoma (some of them marked with yellow arrows in the schematic image, Fig. 3.**4b**) and the areas of the mucinous cancer (corresponding to the blue-colored area in the schematic image) are well seen in the large histologic section. The tumor infiltrated the pericolic fatty tissue. The cancer exhibited obvious intratumoral heterogeneity, as demonstrated in Figure 3.**4a**, which shows a microscopic detail from the area marked with the red rectangle in Figure 3.**4b**. Mucinous carcinoma in the colorectum is defined as a cancer with dominating mucinous structures (more than 50% of the tumor). The large histologic section allows proper assessment of the proportions of different tumor types in cases of heterogeneous tumors, and assists in proper tumor typing. It also helps in appreciating the difficulties in obtaining biopsies representative of the invasive part of the tumor, as in the present case.

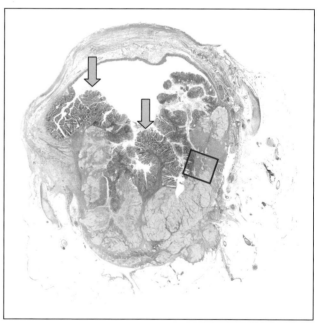

Fig. 3.**4b** Schematic guide to the morphologic details in the large section in Fig. 3.**4**.

### Practical points

- Inclusion of a transection of the entire tumor is a further advantage of large histologic sections, as the proportions of different tumor parts can be determined and heterogeneous tumors can be properly typed.

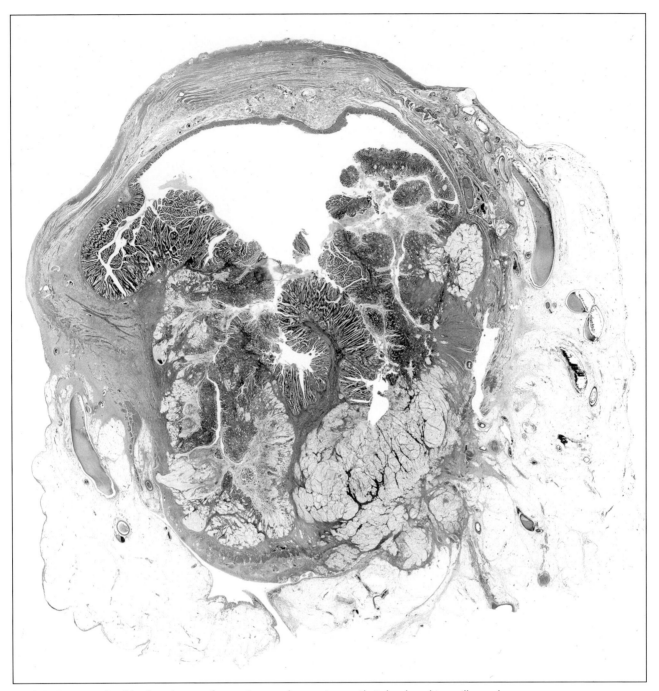

Fig. 3.**4**   Large-section histology image of a mucinous colon carcinoma that developed in a villous adenoma.

## Case 3.5 Invasive Rectal Carcinoma, Dukes C

**Patient data:** 72-year-old woman with anemia. A large malignant lesion was found endoscopically 7 cm from the anus in her rectum. The diagnosis of invasive carcinoma was made on endoscopic biopsy.

**Surgical treatment:** Mesorectal resection, no preoperative irradiation.

**Specimen:** 18-cm-long rectum with a tumor 6 cm in diameter and 2 cm from the distal margin.

**Histopathologic diagnosis:** Moderately differentiated rectal adenocarcinoma infiltrating through the lamina muscularis propria into the pericolic tissue. Four of the 15 examined lymph nodes contained metastases. In addition, isolated tumor foci were found in the perirectal tissue. Radical excision, mesorectal margin 4 mm.

**TNM stage:** IIIC (T3N2M0V2), Dukes C.

**Follow-up:** 14 months, no signs of disease recurrence.

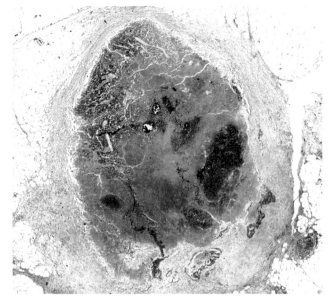

Fig. 3.**5 a**

The large histologic section in Figure 3.**5** demonstrates an invasive carcinoma (corresponding to the red-colored area in the schematic image, Fig. 3.**5 d**), the rest of the tumor being tubulovillous adenoma filling the lumen of the large intestine. An enlarged, tumor-containing, necrotic lymph node is seen on the left upper edge of the image marked with the blue rectangle in Figure 3.**5 d** and is histologically magnified in Figure 3.**5 a**. Isolated foci of infiltrating tumor tissue without histologic evidence of residual lymph node structures in their surroundings are also seen in the mesorectum (partly marked in red and indicated with a blue double arrow in Fig. 3.**5 d**; magnified microscopically in Fig. 3.**5 b**). According to the TNM classification, if the foci have the round form and smooth contour of a lymph node, they should be classified as lymph node metastases. If they are irregular, as in this case, they should be classified as vascular invasion (V1 if seen only microscopically, V2 if seen upon examination with the naked eye). The isolated tumor foci should also influence the measurement of the surgical margin, as indicated with the blue double arrow in Figure 3.**5 d**. In this case, additional lymph nodes are seen in the large section, one of them, marked with the yellow arrow, containing metastasis in the subcapsular sinus (Fig. 3.**5 c**, upper edge of the image).

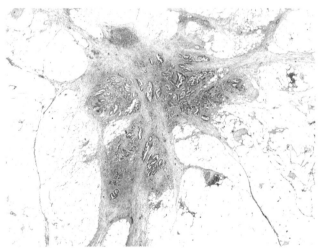

Fig. 3.**5 b**

### Practical points

- Large histologic sections allow examination of a large area of the mesorectum, and thus are an ideal tool for detecting isolated tumor foci in the fatty tissue.
- The isolated tumor foci, depending on their form, should be classified either as lymph node metastasis or as vascular invasion. These foci also influence the status of the surgical margins.

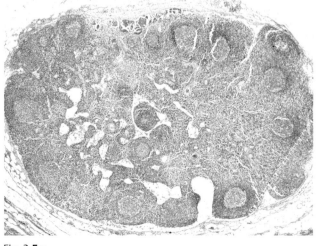

Fig. 3.**5 c**

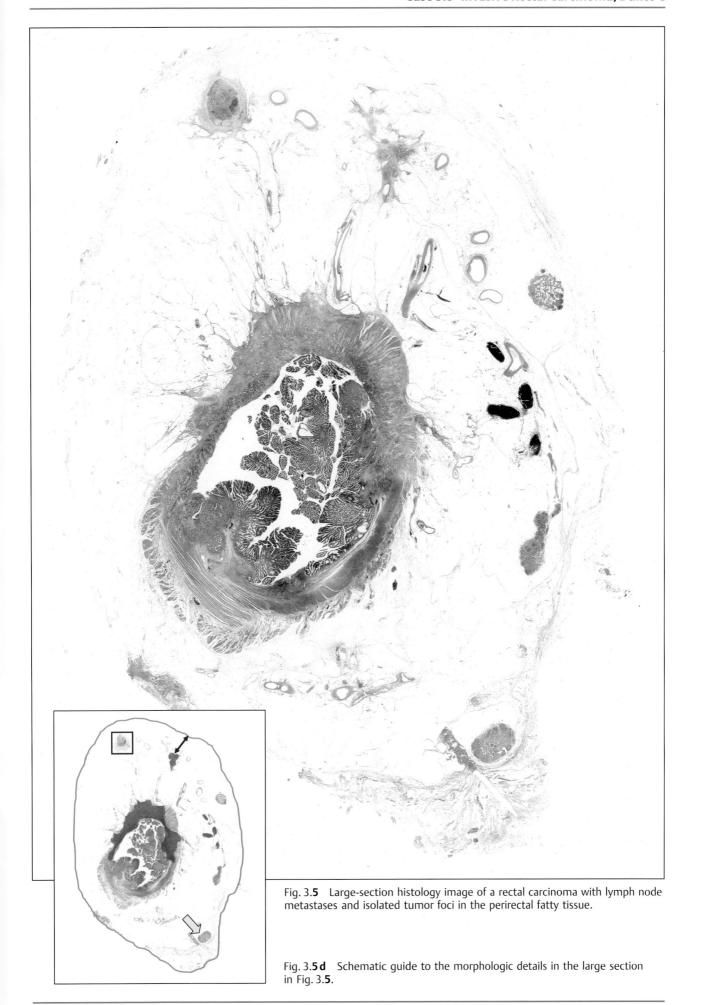

Fig. 3.**5**   Large-section histology image of a rectal carcinoma with lymph node metastases and isolated tumor foci in the perirectal fatty tissue.

Fig. 3.**5 d**   Schematic guide to the morphologic details in the large section in Fig. 3.**5**.

## Case 3.6 Advanced Colon Carcinoma

**Patient data:** 68-year-old woman with subileus and a large palpable tumor in the cecal region.

**Surgical treatment:** Right hemicolectomy, no preoperative irradiation.

**Specimen:** 24-cm-long segment of the colon and an 11-cm part of the terminal ileum with a 5 cm in diameter exophytic tumor in the vicinity of the ileocecal valve; free margins, large palpable nodes in the mesenterium.

**Histopathologic diagnosis:** Moderately differentiated adenocarcinoma infiltrating through the lamina muscularis propria into the pericolic tissue; 26 of the 31 examined lymph nodes contained metastases. In addition, isolated tumor foci were found in the pericolic tissue. Vascular invasion and infiltration of the serosal surface were also evidenced.

**TNM stage:** IIIC (T3N2M0V1), Dukes C.

**Follow-up:** The patient died of the disease 17 months after the operation.

The large histologic section in Figure 3.**6** is very informative as it demonstrates the large exophytic and infiltrating carcinoma in the posterior parts of the cecum (corresponding to the red-colored area in the schematic image, Fig. 3.**6c**) together with a large area of the mesocolon. The tumor infiltrated the intestinal wall and the pericolic fatty tissue, partly forming continuous extensions, partly forming isolated tumor foci (also red-colored in Fig. 3.**6c**) lacking any connection with the main tumor mass. Some of the isolated tumor foci (marked with arrows in Fig. 3.**6c**) are round or oval shaped and have smooth contours. One of them (marked with the yellow arrow) is magnified in Figure 3.**6a**. This lesion represents a borderline structure between a metastatic lymph node and an isolated round tumor focus, as only a minimal rest of the lymphoid tissue is present in the central part of the lesion. However, this borderline image justifies classification of the smooth-contoured isolated tumor foci as lymph node metastases. Figure 3.**6b** is a microscopic magnification of the area of the blue rectangle in Figure 3.**6c** and demonstrates an irregular, isolated tumor focus partially with vascular invasion. Several enlarged lymph nodes containing metastatic tumor structures are also seen (green-colored in Fig. 3.**6c**).

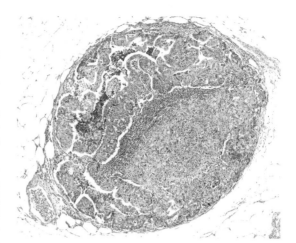

Fig. 3.**6a**

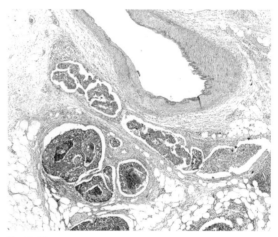

Fig. 3.**6b**

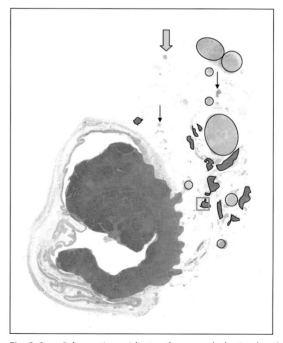

Fig. 3.**6c** Schematic guide to the morphologic details in the large section in Fig. 3.**6**.

### Practical points

- Isolated tumor foci in the mesocolon should be classified as lymph node metastasis if exhibiting a round shape and smooth contours similar to a lymph node.
- Isolated tumor foci with an irregular shape indicate a high probability of vascular invasion.

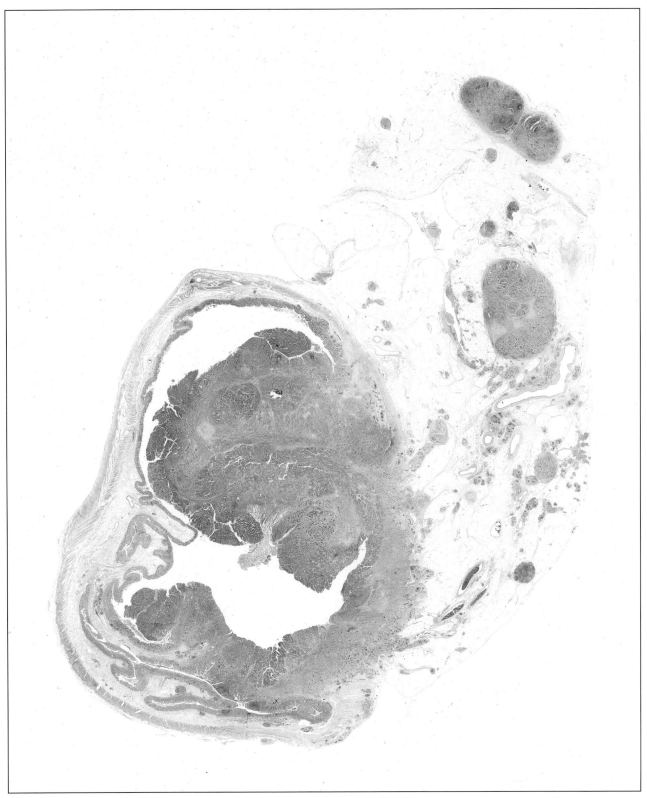

Fig. 3.6  Large-section histology image of an advanced colon carcinoma with lymph nodes metastases and isolated tumor foci in the pericolic fatty tissue.

## Case 3.7 Rectal Carcinoma with Vascular Invasion

**Patient data:** 54-year-old woman with rectal bleeding. Endoscopically, a large, partly ulcerated tumor was seen in her rectum, 10 cm from the anus. A diagnosis of adenocarcinoma was made on endoscopic biopsy. The preoperative radiological work-up revealed metastases in her liver.
**Surgical treatment:** Mesorectal resection, no preoperative irradiation.
**Specimen:** 18-cm-long rectum with a 6 cm in diameter tumor, 4 cm from the distal margin.
**Histopathologic diagnosis:** Moderately differentiated adenocarcinoma infiltrating the lamina muscularis propria. One of the 12 examined lymph nodes contained metastasis. Vascular invasion.
**TNM stage:** IV (T2N1M1V1), Dukes C.
**Follow-up:** 8 months, no signs of recurrence.

The carcinoma demonstrated in the large section in Figure 3.**7** infiltrated almost the whole circumference of the rectum. However, it respected the borders of the lamina muscularis propria and, as such, it could be an early carcinoma with excellent prognosis. Unfortunately, the cancer structures had found a way to invade large vascular spaces (indicated by arrows in the schematic image, Fig. 3.**7d**), one of which (indicated by the orange arrow) is magnified in Figure 3.**7a–c**. These images show a larger vein with a thrombus containing structures of the infiltrating cancer. Vascular invasion is a negative prognostic factor even if the cancer is locally radically excised. Note the wide free mesorectal/circumferential surgical margin.

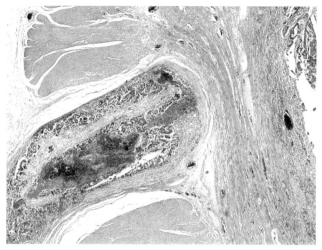

Fig. 3.**7a**

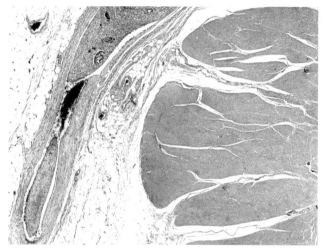

Fig. 3.**7b**

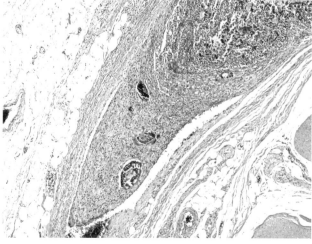

**Practical points**

- Large histologic sections allow examination of a large area of the mesorectum/mesocolon, and make it easier to find and document the presence of vascular invasion, even if it is macroscopically not detectable.

Fig. 3.**7c**

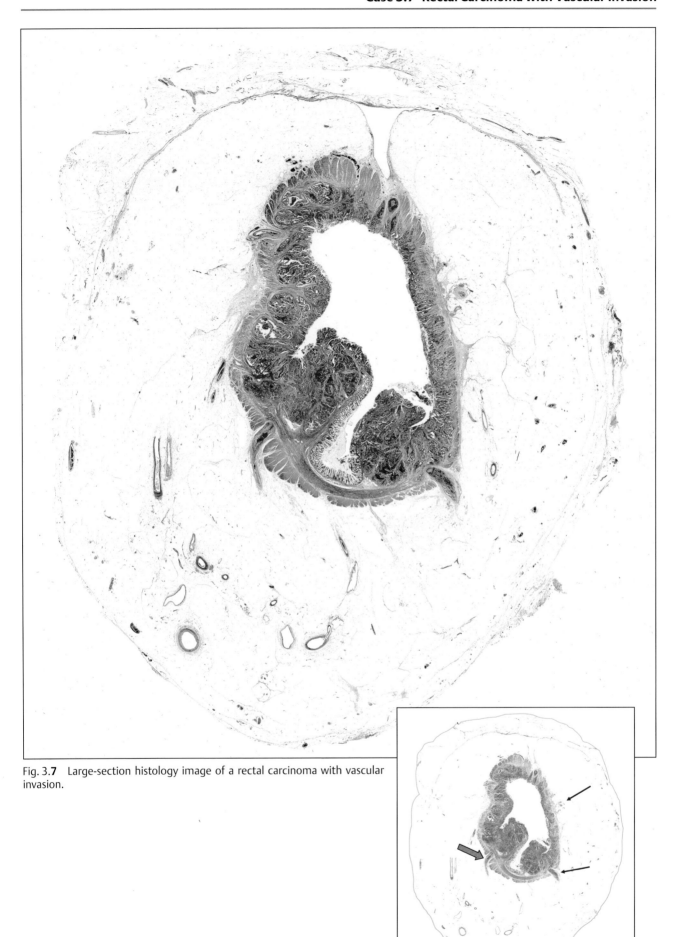

Fig. 3.**7** Large-section histology image of a rectal carcinoma with vascular invasion.

Fig. 3.**7 d** Schematic guide to the morphologic details in the large section in Fig. 3.**7**.

## Case 3.8 Rectal Carcinoma with Vascular Invasion

**Patient data:** 70-year-old man with pain in the thoracic spine. Upon radiological verification of bone metastases, a rectal tumor was detected on digital rectal examination. Endoscopically, a large, partly ulcerated tumor was seen in the rectum, 5 cm from the anus. A diagnosis of adenocarcinoma was made on endoscopic biopsy.

**Surgical treatment:** Rectosigmoidal resection, no preoperative irradiation.

**Specimen:** 40-cm-long rectosigmoideum with a tumor 5 cm in diameter and 4 cm from the distal margin.

**Histopathologic diagnosis:** Moderately differentiated adenocarcinoma infiltrating the lamina muscularis propria and the perirectal fatty tissue. Ten of the 12 examined lymph nodes contained metastasis. Macroscopic and microscopic vascular invasion.

**TNM stage:** IV (T3N2M1V2), Dukes C.

**Follow-up:** The patient died of the disease 4 months after the operation.

The tumor demonstrated in the large histologic section in Figure 3.**8** exhibited an obvious affinity to invade vascular spaces. This explains the discontinuous spread of the tumor through the muscular coat of the rectum and in the mesorectum, as indicated with red-colored areas in the schematic image (Fig. 3.**8 d**). Already in the muscular wall, tumor cells could be found in the vascular lumina. One such area (corresponding to the green rectangle in Fig. 3.**8 d**) is microscopically magnified in Figure 3.**8 a**. Several large vascular spaces were also invaded by tumor structures in the mesorectum, as demonstrated in Figure 3.**8 b**, which represents a magnified image of the area of the red rectangle in Figure 3.**8 d**. Already on macroscopic examination, a large dilated vein containing tumor tissue in a thrombus was seen. A part of it is microscopically magnified in Figure 3.**8 c**. The vein is indicated with the yellow arrow in the schematic image. Macroscopically seen vascular invasion is classified as category V2 in the TNM classification. This type of tumor spread is a negative morphologic prognostic factor.

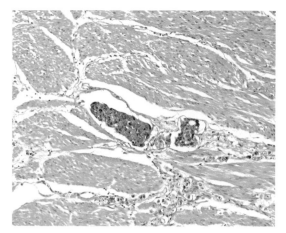

Fig. 3.**8 a**

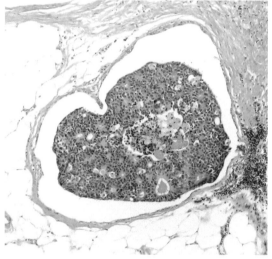

Fig. 3.**8 b**

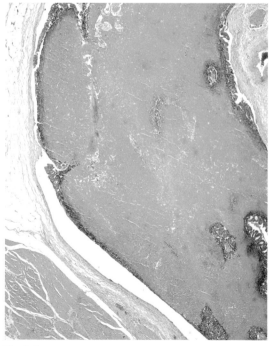

### Practical points

- Macroscopic and microscopic vascular invasion is usually associated with metastatic tumor spread and an unfavorable prognosis.

Fig. 3.**8 c**

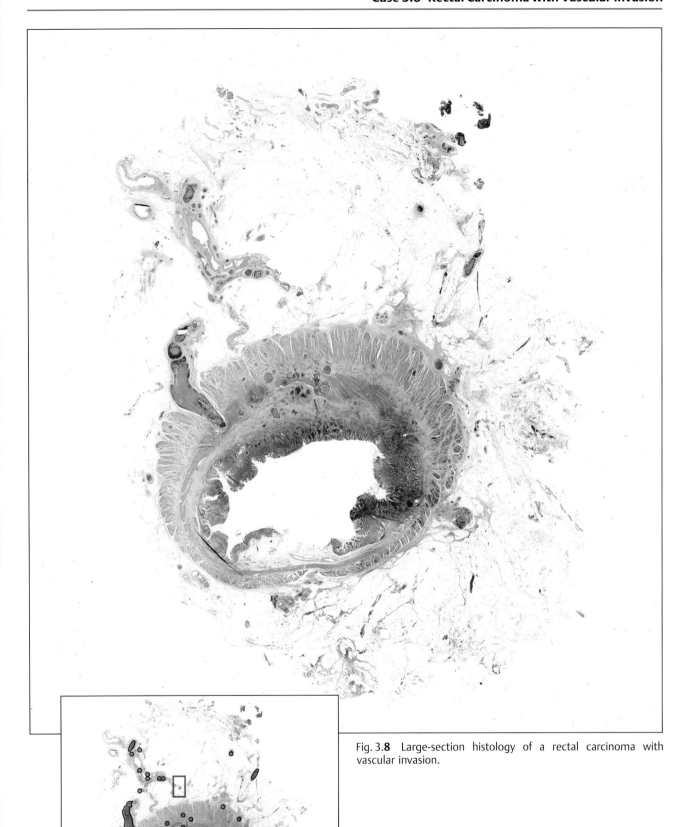

Fig. 3.8 Large-section histology of a rectal carcinoma with vascular invasion.

Fig. 3.8 d Schematic guide to the morphologic details in the large section in Fig. 3.8.

## Case 3.9 Colon Carcinoma with Periarterial Invasion and Lymph Node Metastasis

**Patient data:** 77-year-old man with rectal bleeding. Endoscopically, a stenotic segment in sigmoid colon was seen approximately 30 cm from the anus. A diagnosis of adenocarcinoma was made on endoscopic biopsy.
**Surgical treatment:** Left hemicolectomy, no preoperative irradiation.
**Specimen:** 60-cm-long segment of the colon with a 6 × 5-cm tumor, 10 cm from the proximal margin.
**Histopathologic diagnosis:** Moderately differentiated adenocarcinoma infiltrating through the lamina muscularis propria into the perirectal fatty tissue. Ten of the 13 examined lymph nodes contained metastasis. Microscopic vascular engagement.
**TNM stage:** IIIC (T3N2M0V1), Dukes C.
**Follow-up:** 24 months, no signs of disease recurrence.

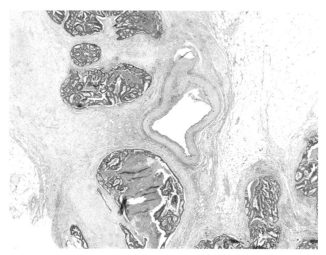

Fig. 3.**9a**

The large histological section in Figure 3.**9** demonstrates periarterial spread of an invasive colon carcinoma. The areas corresponding to tumor tissue in the colon and to the isolated tumor foci around the artery are green-colored in the schematic image (Fig. 3.**9d**). The intimate relationship of the tumor structures and the arterial wall (red-colored structures in Fig. 3.**9d**) is evident in the large section and is further illustrated in Figure 3.**9a, b**. Figure 3.**9a** (magnified area of the red rectangle in Fig. 3.**9d**) illustrates the minimal distance between a branch of the artery and the tumor structures. Figure 3.**9b** is a microscopic magnification from the area corresponding to the blue rectangle in the schematic image. The wall of the artery is demonstrated on the left side of the image and an isolated island of tumor tissue on the right side. The irregular contours of the isolated tumor foci in the vicinity of the artery suggest that they represent vascular invasion. Some of the isolated foci, however, have smooth contours. One of them (marked with the yellow rectangle in Fig. 3.**9d** and magnified in Fig. 3.**9c**) is surrounded by structures of a partly destroyed lymph node and is a lymph node metastasis.

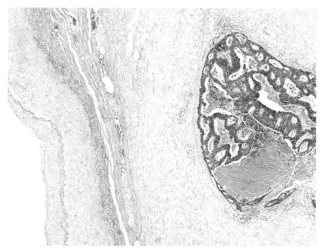

Fig. 3.**9b**

### Practical points

- The large histologic section allows examination of an extensive area of the mesorectum/mesocolon, making it easier to find and document the presence of metastatic lymph nodes, vascular invasion, and, as in this particular case, perivascular invasion.
- The pattern of invasion is clearly demonstrated in relation to the structures of the mesocolon.

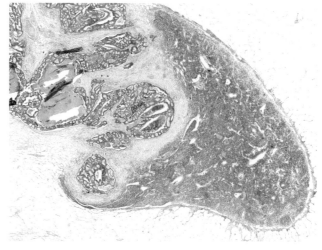

Fig. 3.**9c**

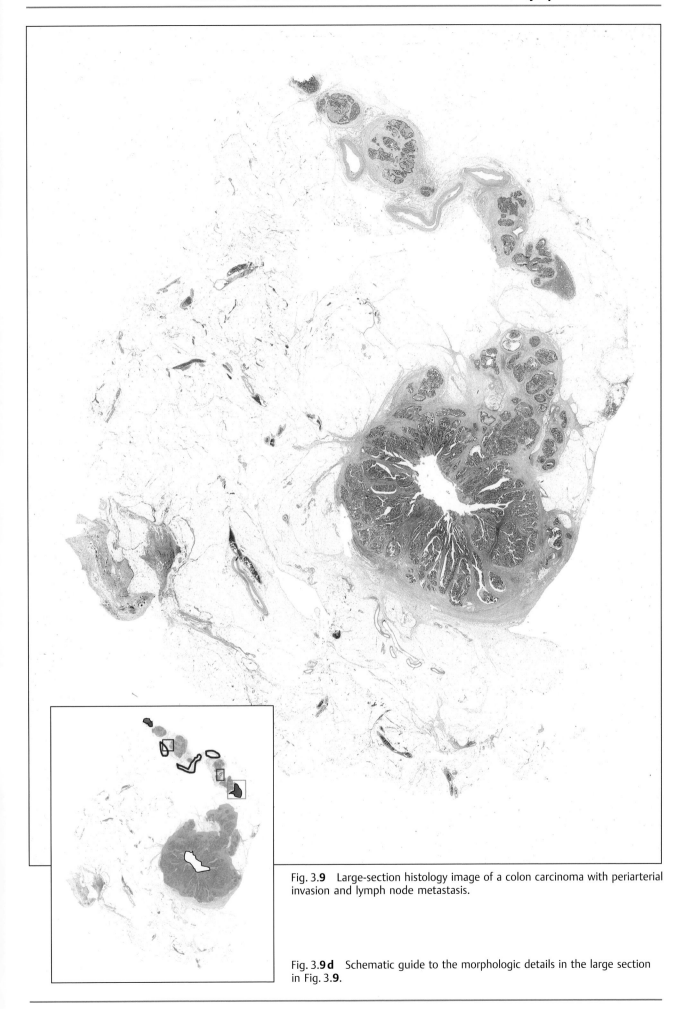

Fig. 3.**9**   Large-section histology image of a colon carcinoma with periarterial invasion and lymph node metastasis.

Fig. 3.**9 d**   Schematic guide to the morphologic details in the large section in Fig. 3.**9**.

## Case 3.10 Mucinous Colon Carcinoma with Lymph Node Metastasis

**Patient data:** 88-year-old woman with abdominal pain. Endoscopically, an exophytic tumor was seen in the sigmoid colon. No preoperative biopsy was performed.
**Surgical treatment:** Left hemicolectomy, no preoperative irradiation.
**Specimen:** 65-cm-long colon segment centrally with a 9 × 9-cm tumor.
**Histopathologic diagnosis:** Well-differentiated mucinous adenocarcinoma infiltrating the lamina muscularis propria and the subserosa on the ventral surface. Three of the 16 examined lymph nodes contained metastasis. Microscopic vascular engagement.
**TNM stage:** IIIB (T3N1M0V1), Dukes C.
**Follow-up:** 9 months, no signs of disease recurrence.

The large histologic section in Figure 3.**10** demonstrates a mucinous colon carcinoma that has developed in a villous adenoma. The rests of the adenoma cover approximately the mesocolic half of the circumference of the bowel wall, while the invasive carcinoma covers the anterior part. The tissue of the mucinous carcinoma corresponds to the blue-colored area in the schematic image (Fig. 3.**10c**). Some structures of the villous adenoma are indicated with yellow arrows. The level of invasion is well seen. Several lymph nodes are present in the mesenterium; one of them (marked with the red rectangle in Fig. 3.**10c**) contained metastasis and is histologically magnified in Figure 3.**10a**. Further magnification of the metastatic mucinous carcinoma in this lymph node is seen in Figure 3.**10b** (alcian-blue stain demonstrating mucin).

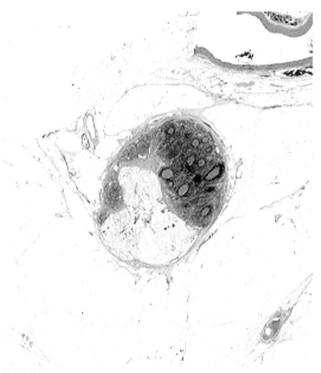

Fig. 3.**10a**

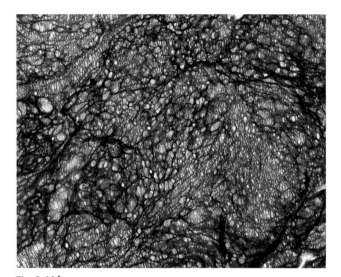

Fig. 3.**10b**

### Practical points

- A single large histologic section may allow proper classification of the tumor and staging of the disease at the same time, as it may include several lymph nodes in addition to a representative section of the primary tumor.

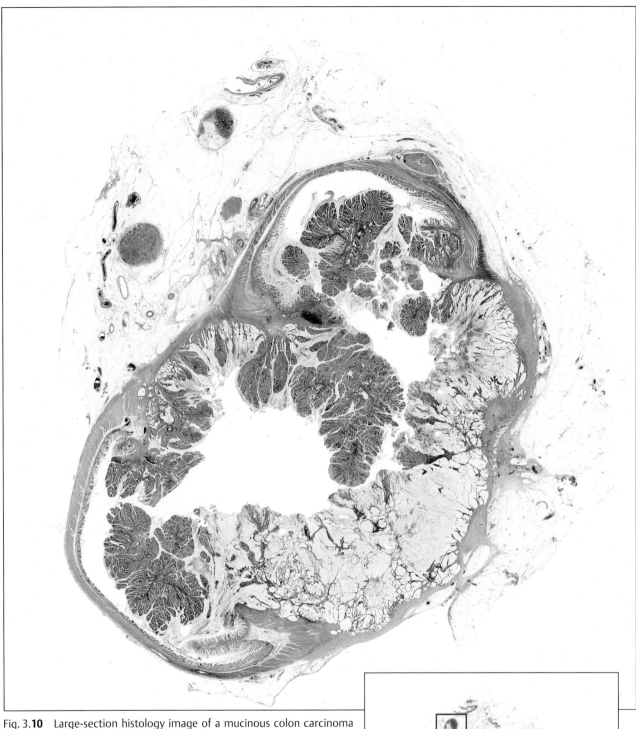

Fig. 3.**10**  Large-section histology image of a mucinous colon carcinoma with lymph node metastasis.

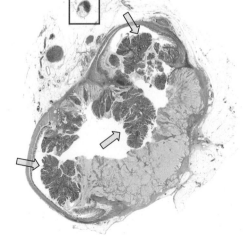

Fig. 3.**10 c**  Schematic guide to the morphologic details in the large section in Fig. 3.**10**.

## Case 3.11 Advanced Mucinous Cancer

**Patient data:** 73-year-old woman with rectal bleeding. Endoscopically, a large somewhat exophytic tumor was seen in her rectum, 5 cm from the anus. No preoperative biopsy was performed.
**Surgical treatment:** Mesorectal resection, no preoperative irradiation.
**Specimen:** 20-cm-long rectum with a tumor 5 cm in diameter and 4 cm from the distal margin.
**Histopathologic diagnosis:** Well-differentiated mucinous adenocarcinoma infiltrating through the lamina muscularis propria. Three of the 16 examined lymph nodes contained metastasis. Radical excision.
**TNM stage:** IIIB (T3N1M0), Dukes C.
**Follow-up:** 31 months, no signs of disease recurrence.

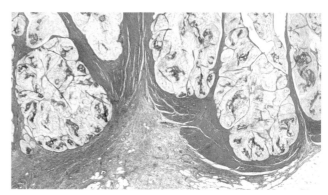

Fig. 3.**11 a**

The mucinous carcinoma demonstrated in Figure 3.**11** seemingly respected the border of the lamina muscularis propria, as seen on macroscopic examination and in the large histologic section. However, closer examination of the tumor contours towards the mesorectum reveals invasion into the fatty tissue. Magnification (Fig. 3.**11 a**) of the area corresponding to the red rectangle in Figure 3.**11 c** also demonstrates the absence of smooth muscle cells under the mucinous tumor structures on the left side of the image (compared to the right side of the image, where the smooth muscles bundles are preserved). One of the lymph nodes in the mesorectum is filled with metastasis of the mucinous tumor. Figure 3.**11 b** is a microscopic magnification of the area of the blue rectangle in the schematic image and demonstrates the interface of a lymph node free of metastasis and the lymph node containing metastasis of the mucinous cancer. The area of primary and metastatic tumor tissue is blue-colored in the schematic image (Fig. 3.**11 c**). Note the artery and the vein (marked with yellow arrows in the lowest part of the image).

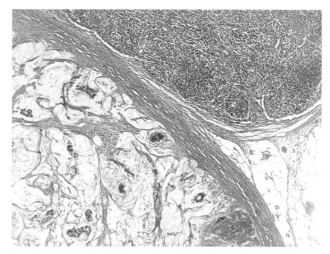

Fig. 3.**11 b**

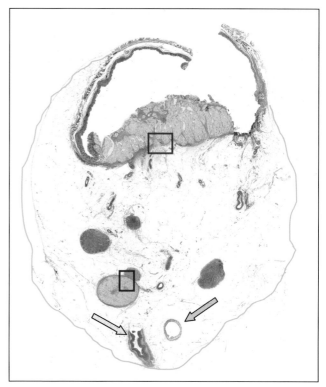

Fig. 3.**11 c**   Schematic guide to the morphologic details in the large section in Fig. 3.**11**.

### Practical points

- The large histologic section allows examination of an extensive area of the mesorectum/mesocolon, making it easier to find and document the presence of metastatic lymph nodes in relation to the primary tumor.

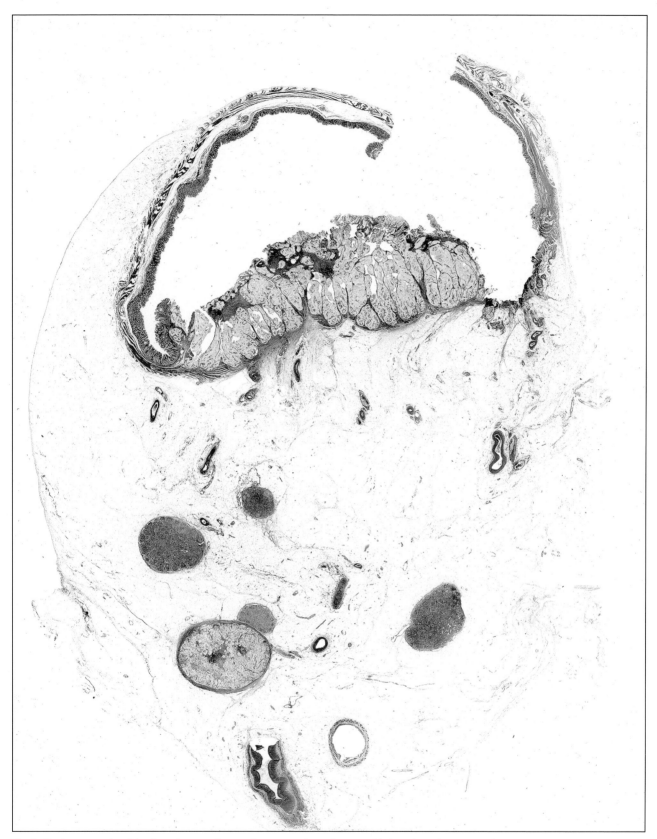

Fig. 3.**11**  Large-section histology image of a mucinous rectal carcinoma with lymph node metastasis.

## Case 3.12 Advanced Mucinous Carcinoma of the Colon with Lymph Node Metastasis and Vascular Invasion

**Patient data:** 71-year-old man presenting with abdominal pain. Endoscopically, a large tumor mass was seen in the sigmoid colon. The diagnosis of invasive mucinous carcinoma was made on preoperative biopsy.
**Surgical treatment:** Subtotal colectomy, no preoperative irradiation.
**Specimen:** 65-cm-long segment of the large intestine with an 8 × 8-cm exophytic tumor in the sigmoidal part, 12 cm from the distal margin.
**Histopathologic diagnosis:** Mucinous carcinoma, low grade, infiltrating beyond the lamina muscularis propria, 9 of the 9 examined lymph nodes contained metastasis. Radical excision.
**TNM stage:** IIIC (T3N2M0V1), Dukes C.
**Follow-up:** Died of metastatic colon carcinoma 12 months after the operation.

The large section in Figure 3.**12** shows an advanced mucinous carcinoma of the colon infiltrating all the layers of the intestinal wall and the pericolic fatty tissue. The tumor tissue is indicated with a transparent blue area in the schematic image (Fig. 3.**12c**) and shows that, besides the large mass of mucinous cancer within the bowel wall and the continuous extension of the tumor into the fatty tissue, there are also isolated tumor foci in the mesenterium. The isolated foci with smooth contours and round/oval forms are enlarged lymph nodes (indicated by yellow arrows in Fig. 3.**12c**), containing metastases of the mucinous cancer. Figure 3.**12a** is a magnification of a metastatic lymph node with a minimal rest of lymphoid tissue in the lower edge of the node. The irregular, isolated tumor foci in the fatty tissue (indicated with the orange arrows) are outside the lymph nodes and some of them are in an intimate relation to large blood vessels. Figure 3.**12b** demonstrates one such isolated tumor focus in the immediate vicinity of a larger vessel (corresponding to the area indicated with the red rectangle in the schematic image, Fig. 3.**12c**). As demonstrated before, these isolated tumor foci represent discontinuous spread of the tumor. When exhibiting smooth contours, they are classified as lymph node metastases according to the TNM classification, while when irregular, they indicate a high probability of vascular invasion.

**Practical points**

- Mucinous colorectal carcinomas may exhibit an aggressive biological behavior, even if they are well-differentiated.
- Isolated tumor foci in the vicinity of blood vessels indicate a high probability of vascular invasion and represent a negative prognostic parameter.

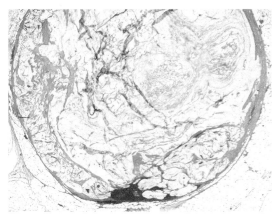

Fig. 3.**12a**

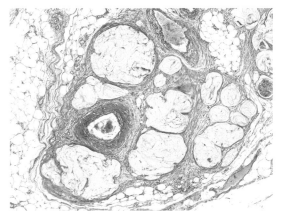

Fig. 3.**12b**

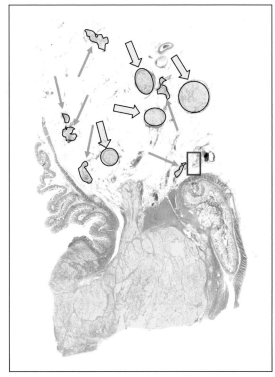

Fig. 3.**12c** Schematic guide to the morphologic details in the large section in Fig. 3.**12**.

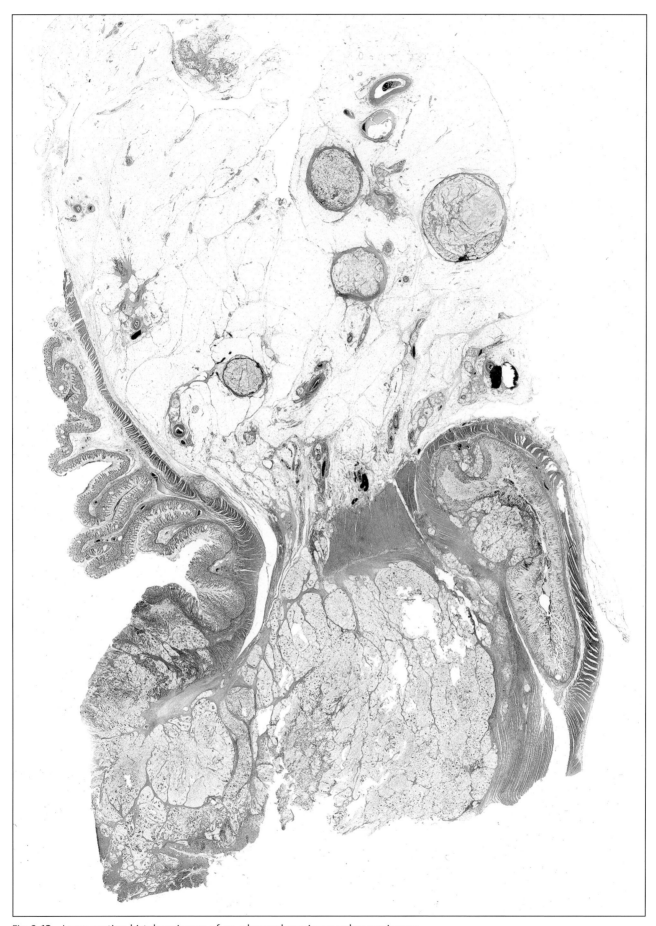

Fig. 3.**12**  Large-section histology image of an advanced mucinous colon carcinoma.

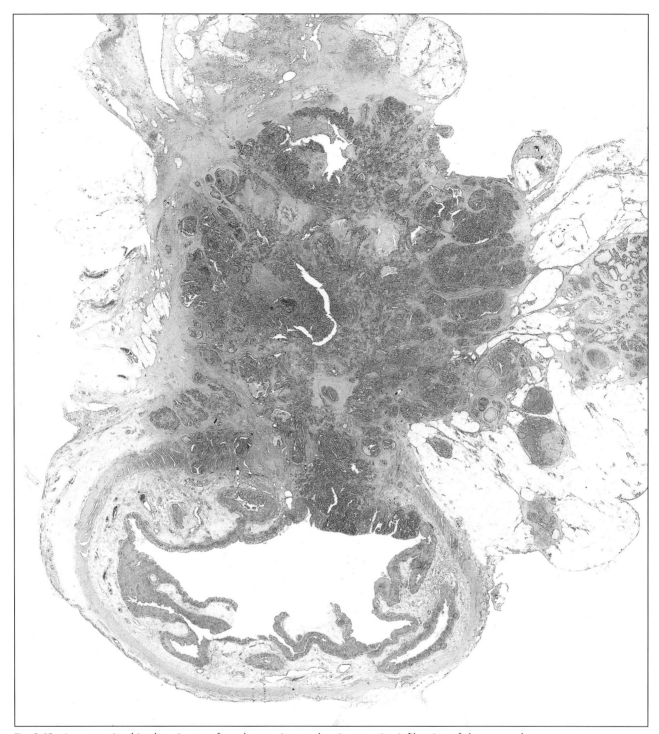

Fig. 3.**13**  Large-section histology image of a colon carcinoma showing massive infiltration of the mesocolon.

## Cases 3.13 and 3.14  Massive Infiltration of the Mesocolon

The primary colon carcinomas demonstrated in the large histologic sections in Figures 3.**13 and** 3.**14** caused only a minor elevation of the luminal surface of the intestine. The infiltrative portions of the tumors were disproportionately larger than the small intraintestinal part. The massive infiltrate in the mesocolon reached the surface of the serosa.

Case 3.13 represents a carcinoma with only focal necrosis, while extensive necrosis of the tumor mass in the mesenterium, as in Case 3.14, may cause formation of a pseudolumen. Note the metastatic lymph node and the numerous isolated tumor foci in the fatty tissue in both large sections.

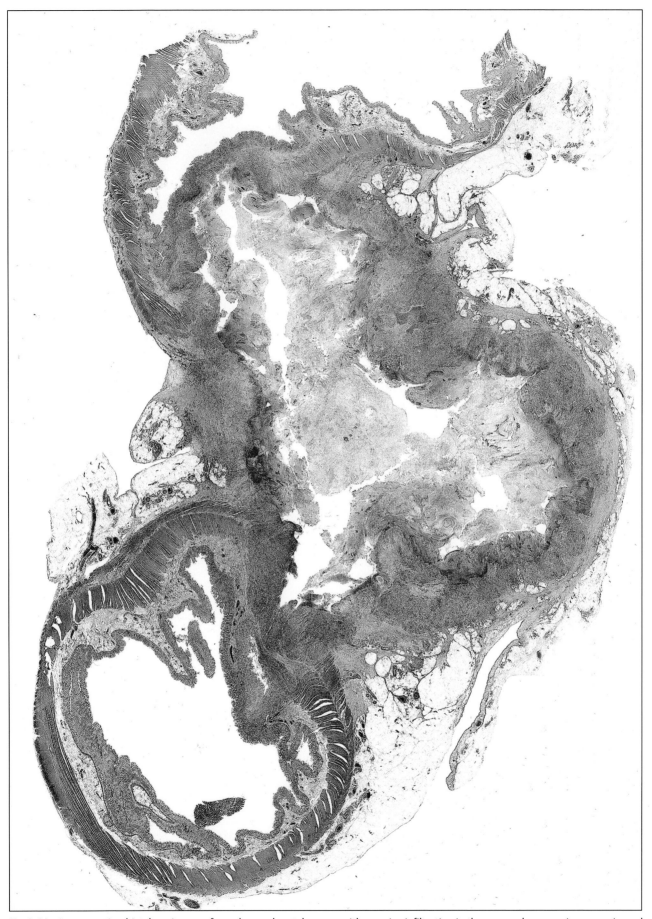

Fig. 3.**14**  Large-section histology image of an advanced rectal cancer with massive infiltration in the mesocolon, massive necrosis, and a pseudolumen.

## Case 3.15 Advanced Rectal Carcinoma Invading the Serosal Surface

**Patient data:** 80-year-old woman presenting with rectal bleeding. Endoscopically, an ulcerated tumor was seen on the border of the rectum and sigmoid colon. The diagnosis of invasive carcinoma was made on endoscopic biopsy.

**Surgical treatment:** Rectosigmoidal resection, no preoperative irradiation.

**Specimen:** 16-cm-long segment of the large intestine with a 4 × 5-cm ulcerated tumor, 6 cm from the distal margin.

**Histopathologic diagnosis:** Moderately differentiated adenocarcinoma infiltrating beyond the lamina muscularis propria. Isolated tumor foci in the mesenterium. Serosal involvement. Four of the 14 examined lymph nodes contained metastasis.

**TNM stage:** IIIc (T4N2M0), Dukes C

**Follow-up:** 10 months, no signs of disease recurrence.

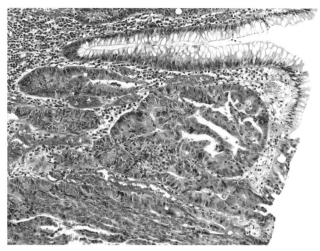

Fig. 3.**15 a**

The large section in Figure 3.**15** demonstrates an advanced carcinoma infiltrating through all the layers of the intestinal wall into the pericolic fatty tissue. The area corresponding to the yellow rectangle in the schematic image (Fig. 3.**15 d**) is microscopically magnified in Figure 3.**15 a** and demonstrates the abrupt transition of the normal epithelium into malignant tissue. The tumor infiltrated the serosal surface in its invaginated part (demonstrated on the left side of the image, marked with the blue arrow in Fig. 3.**15 d** and magnified in Fig. 3.**15 b**). Figure 3.**15 c** represents a magnification of an isolated tumor focus around a large blood vessel (corresponding to the area of the red rectangle in Fig. 3.**15 d**). According to the TNM classification, tumors infiltrating the serosal surface are classified as T4. Narrow spaces in the invaginations of the serosal surface, although difficult to detect on macroscopic examination, may represent a source of „occult" peritoneal spread of the cancer cells. See also Case 3.16.

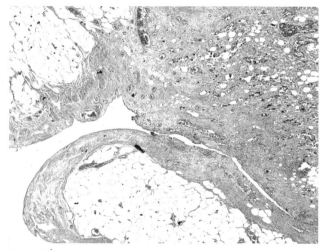

Fig. 3.**15 b**

### Practical points

- By including a transection of the entire specimen, large histologic sections may demonstrate invaginations of the peritoneum following lobulation of the fatty tissue. These narrow spaces may represent source of „occult" peritoneal spread of the cancer cells.

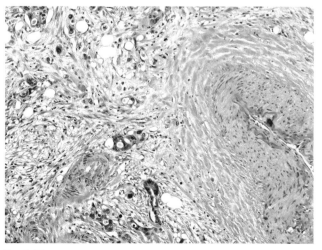

Fig. 3.**15 c**

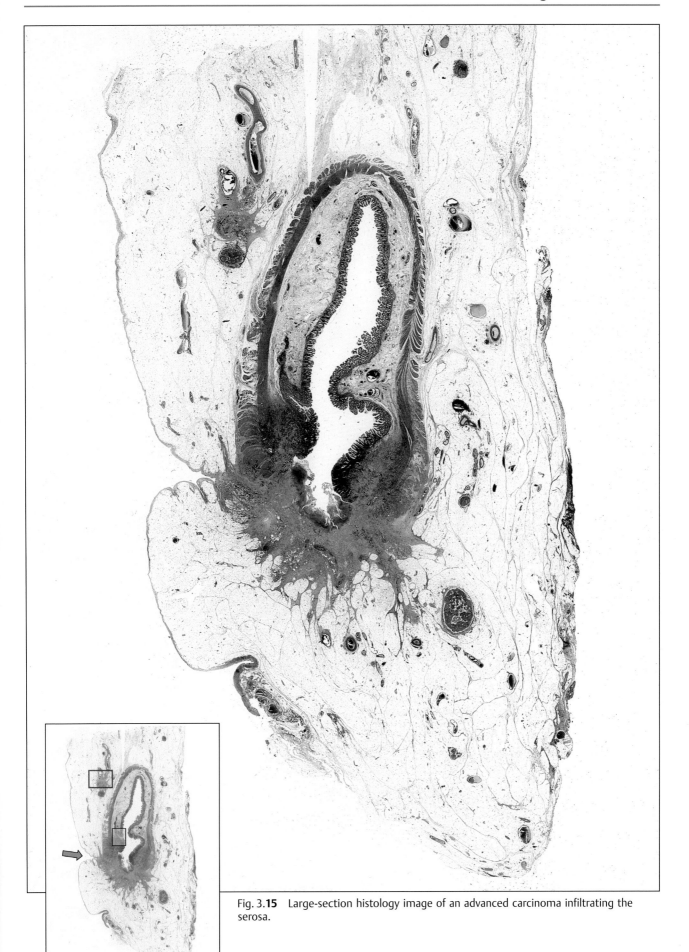

Fig. 3.**15**  Large-section histology image of an advanced carcinoma infiltrating the serosa.

Fig. 3.**15 d**  Schematic guide to the morphologic details in the large section in Fig. 3.**15**.

## Case 3.16 Advanced Colon Carcinoma Causing Intestinal Obstruction

**Patient data:** 86-year-old woman presenting with signs of intestinal obstruction. A stenosing colon carcinoma was seen during laparotomy of the sigmoid colon; liver metastases were also detected.

**Surgical treatment:** Acute sigmoideum resection, needle biopsy of the liver metastases.

**Specimen:** 10-cm-long segment of the large intestine with a 4-cm-long central stenotic part.

**Histopathologic diagnosis:** Moderately differentiated colon adenocarcinoma infiltrating beyond the lamina muscularis propria. Isolated tumor foci in the mesenterium. Serosal involvement. Six of the 9 examined lymph nodes contained metastasis.

**TNM stage:** IV (T4N2M1)

**Follow-up:** 2 months, no signs of disease recurrence.

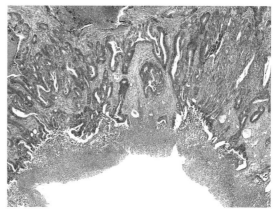

Fig. 3.**16 a**

The large section in Figure 3.**16** demonstrates an advanced colon carcinoma infiltrating through all the layers of the intestinal wall into the pericolic fatty tissue. The tumor tissue is indicated with a transparent red color in the schematic image (Fig. 3.**16 d**). The image also shows a large isolated tumor focus in the mesenterium, corresponding to a metastasis. The lumen of the large intestine is extremely stenotic and is reduced to a narrow channel in the necrotic central part of the tumor. A detail of the necrotic surface of the tumor tissue (corresponding to the green rectangle in Fig. 3.**16 d**) is histologically magnified in Figure 3.**16 a**. The isolated tumor focus in the mesenterium is also magnified (Fig. 3.**16 b**). Figure 3.**16 c** represents a section of the needle biopsy of the liver metastasis, stained immunohistochemically for CDX2, a sensitive marker of tumors of intestinal origin (Tot 2004). Note the preserved liver tissue in the upper part of this image. The contour of the outer surface of the specimen should also be noted as it clearly exhibits invaginations of the serosal surface following lobulation of the fatty tissue. These invaginations are most prominent in the blue-marked segments of the silhouette of the specimen in Figure 3.**16 d**. The narrow spaces may represent a source of „occult" peritoneal spread of the cancer cells.

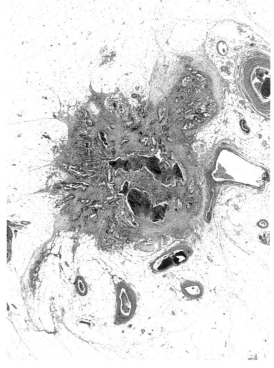

Fig. 3.**16 b**

### Practical points

- Including an entire transection of the intestinal wall containing tumor tissue allows assessment of the intestinal lumen as well.
- In a transection that includes the entire specimen, invaginations of the peritoneum following lobulation of the fatty tissue may be seen. These narrow spaces could represent source of „occult" peritoneal spread of the cancer cells.

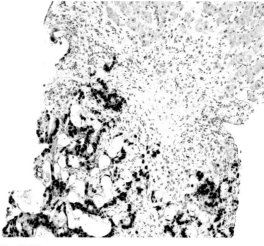

Fig. 3.**16 c**

Fig. 3.**16 d** Schematic guide to the morphologic details in the large section in Fig. 3.**16**.

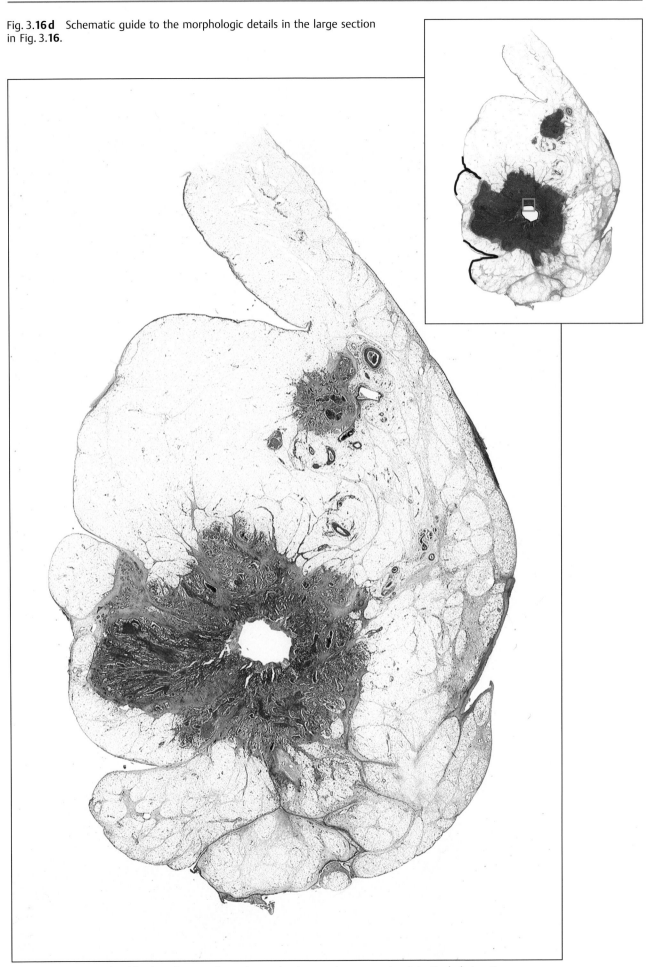

Fig. 3.**16** Large-section histology image of an advanced colon carcinoma causing intestinal obstruction.

## Case 3.17 Colon Carcinoma Causing Subileus

**Patient data:** 80-year-old man presenting with abdominal pain. Endoscopically, a large tumor mass was seen in the sigmoid colon. The diagnosis of invasive carcinoma was made on preoperative biopsy. During the laparotomy, massive peritoneal carcinosis and liver metastases were detected.

**Surgical treatment:** Palliative resection of the sigmoid colon, no preoperative irradiation.

**Specimen:** 18-cm-long segment of the large intestine with a tumorous stenotic part, 4 cm from the nearest margin.

**Histopathologic diagnosis:** Moderately differentiated adenocarcinoma infiltrating beyond the lamina muscularis propria. Five of the 10 examined lymph nodes contained metastasis. Peritoneal metastases. Vascular invasion.

**TNM stage:** IV (T4N2M1V1)

**Follow-up:** Died of metastatic colon carcinoma 1 month after the operation.

The colon carcinoma demonstrated in Figure 3.**17** caused extreme narrowing of the intestinal lumen, leading to sub-occlusion. The tumor infiltrated the entire circumference of the colon and was deeply ulcerated. The red-colored areas in the schematic image (Fig. 3.**17 d**) indicate the tumor tissue in the intestinal wall as well as in the fatty tissue as isolated foci. The narrow lumen is microscopically magnified in Figure 3.**17 a**. Some of the isolated tumor foci (two of them indicated with blue arrows in the schematic image) infiltrated the serosal surface, as also demonstrated microscopically in Figure **17 b**. Some large veins contained tumor tissue (one of them is indicated by the yellow arrow). The smallest lymph node in the specimen, measuring only 1 mm in diameter, contained metastasis. This node is indicated with the red circle in Figure 3.**17 d** and is histologically magnified in Figure 3.**17 c**.

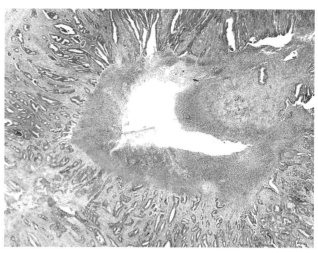

Fig. 3.**17 a**

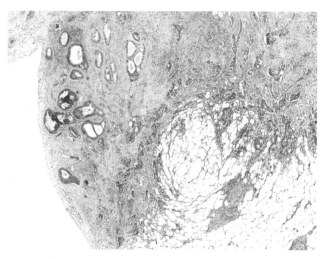

Fig. 3.**17 b**

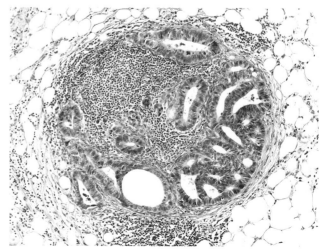

**Practical points**

- The size of the lymph node is not a valuable indicator of the presence or absence of metastasis.

Fig. 3.**17 c**

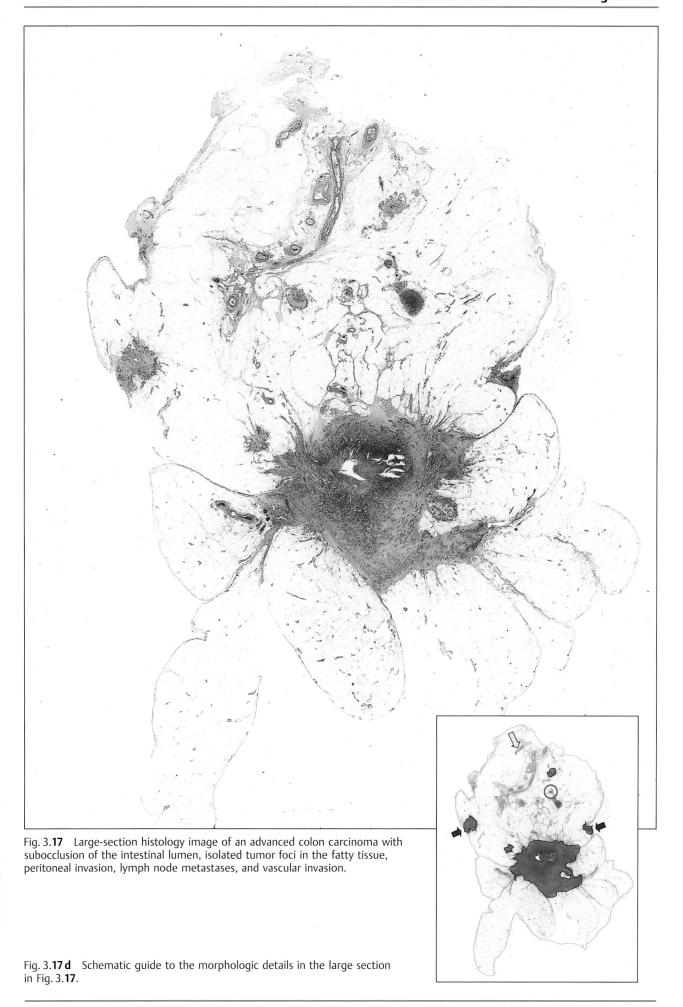

Fig. 3.**17**  Large-section histology image of an advanced colon carcinoma with subocclusion of the intestinal lumen, isolated tumor foci in the fatty tissue, peritoneal invasion, lymph node metastases, and vascular invasion.

Fig. 3.**17 d**  Schematic guide to the morphologic details in the large section in Fig. 3.**17**.

## Case 3.18 Advanced Colon Carcinoma with Lymph Node Metastasis

**Patient data:** 81-year-old male patient presenting with weight loss. Endoscopically, a large tumor was seen in his sigmoid colon. A diagnosis of invasive carcinoma was made on preoperative endoscopic biopsy.

**Surgical treatment:** Left hemicolectomy, no preoperative irradiation.

**Specimen:** 19-cm-long segment of the large intestine with a 4 × 4-cm infiltrating tumor, 8 cm from the distal margin. Extremely enlarged lymph nodes in the mesenterium.

**Histopathologic diagnosis:** Moderately differentiated adenocarcinoma infiltrating beyond the lamina muscularis propria. Three of the 10 examined lymph nodes contained metastasis, radical excision.

**TNM stage:** IIIB (T3N1M0), Dukes C.

**Follow-up:** 18 months, no signs of disease recurrence.

The large histologic section in Figure 3.**18** demonstrates how large the lymph node metastases may be. The metastatic deposits in the two lymph nodes (indicated with yellow- and orange-colored areas in the schematic image, Fig. 3.**18 a**) in this particular case represented a tumor mass that is larger than the primary tumor itself (indicated with the green-colored area in Fig. 3.**18 a**). In the vicinity of the enlarged lymph nodes containing metastases, a small reactive lymph node was found. A part of it is shown in the large section (indicated by the green arrow in Fig. 3.**18 a**). The size of the node is not indicative of metastasis; sometimes the metastatic nodes are considerably enlarged, but very small lymph nodes (as demonstrated in Case 3.17) may also contain metastasis. An inflammatory reaction surrounding the primary tumor was also present.

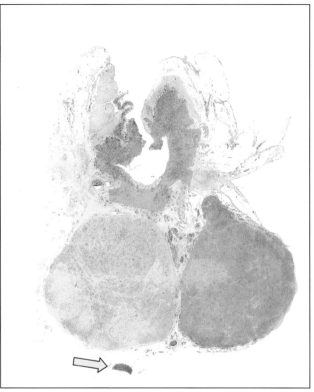

Fig. 3.**18 a** Schematic guide to the morphologic details in the large section in Fig. 3.**18**.

### Practical points

- The tumor mass represented by the lymph node metastases may exceed the mass of the primary tumor.
- Very large metastatic lymph nodes may be accompanied by only slightly enlarged reactive node(s) of normal size within the same specimen.

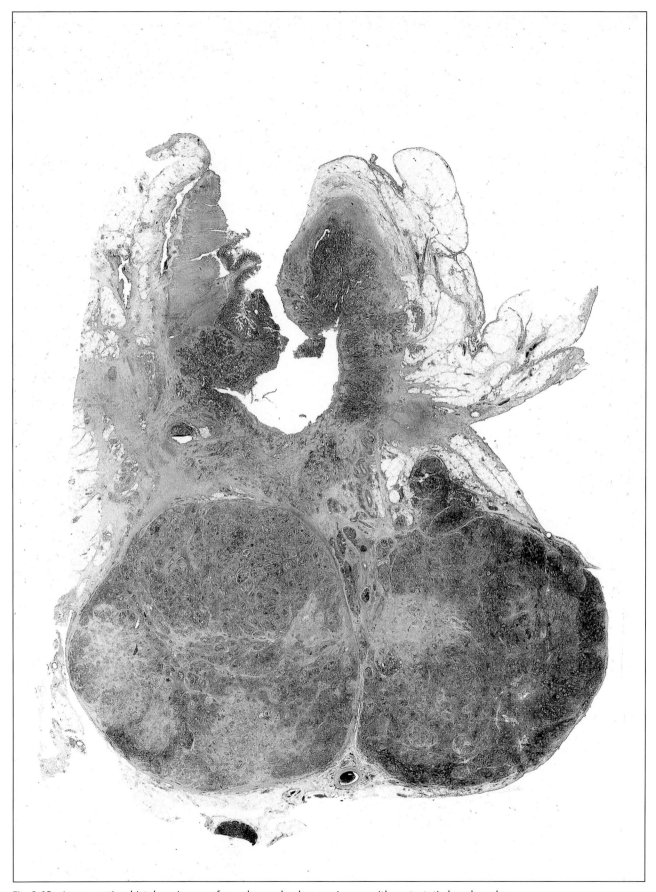

Fig. 3.**18**   Large-section histology image of an advanced colon carcinoma with metastatic lymph nodes.

## Case 3.19 Advanced Colon Carcinoma with Contact Metastasis

**Patient data:** 83-year-old female patient presenting with abdominal pain and palpable tumor in the upper abdomen. During laparotomy, a large tumor was seen in her colon transversum, which was adherent to the abdominal wall. The tumor also infiltrated the wall of the colon descendens.

**Surgical treatment:** Left hemicolectomy, no preoperative irradiation.

**Specimen:** 20-cm-long segment of the large intestine with an 8-cm infiltrating tumor giving contact metastasis to another loop of the large intestine, also resected and present in the specimen. Inflammatory adhesions to the structures of the abdominal wall.

**Histopathologic diagnosis:** Moderately differentiated adenocarcinoma of the colon transversum with contact metastasis into the colon descendens. Four of the 10 examined lymph nodes contained metastasis.

**TNM stage:** IIIC (T4N2M0), Dukes C.

**Follow-up:** 8 months, no signs of disease recurrence.

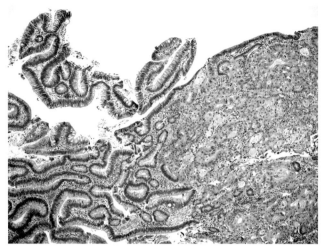

Fig. 3.**19a**

Direct invasion of other segments of the colorectum by way of the serosa indicates category T4 in the TNM classification and represents an unfavorable prognostic factor. This situation is demonstrated in Figure 3.**19**. The large, invasive, mainly mucinous colon carcinoma represented in the large histologic section corresponds to the blue-colored area in the schematic image (Fig. 3.**19d**). The tumor has developed in an adenoma, which is also represented in the large section (marked with the blue arrow in Fig. 3.**19d**). Figure 3.**19a** illustrates the adenoma-carcinoma interface (representing a magnified detail from the area indicated with the yellow arrow in the schematic image). The muscularis propria of the otherwise intact part of the large intestine (upper right corner of the image) is infiltrated by tumor structures. This region of direct invasion into the other intestinal loop (marked with the red rectangle in Fig. 3.**19d**) is microscopically magnified in Figure 3.**19b**. Infiltration of the abdominal wall was also suspected intraoperatively. However, the part of the abdominal muscle at the lower edge of the large-section image is free of invasion. The lymph node in the upper left corner of the image (indicated with the orange rectangle in Fig. 3.**19d**) contained a metastasis, and is magnified in Figure 3.**19c**.

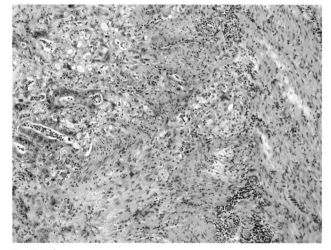

Fig. 3.**19b**

### Practical points

- A single large histologic section may include different regions of the large intestine, which may be of advantage when demonstrating contact metastasis.
- The non-fragmented image in a single large histologic section, including the tumor, the surrounding structures and some structures of the mesocolon, may be sufficient for diagnosing, typing, grading and staging of the represented carcinoma.

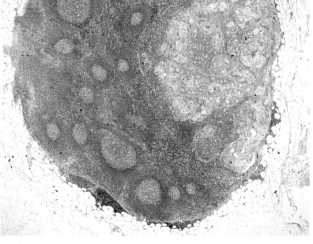

Fig. 3.**19c**

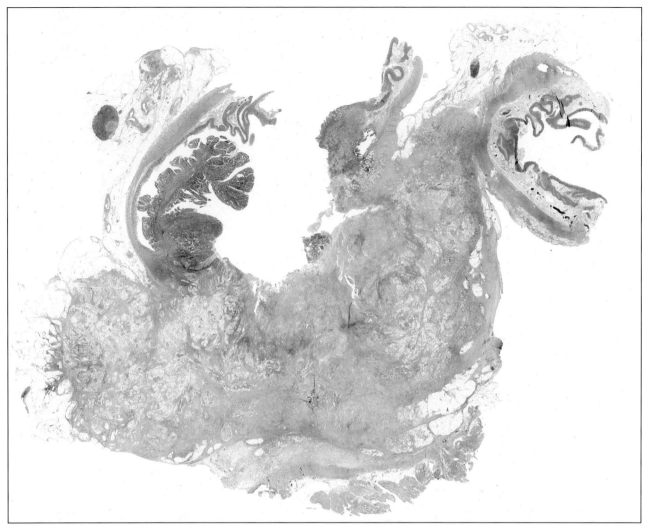

Fig. 3.**19**   Large-section histology image of an advanced colon carcinoma with lymph node metastasis and contact metastasis.

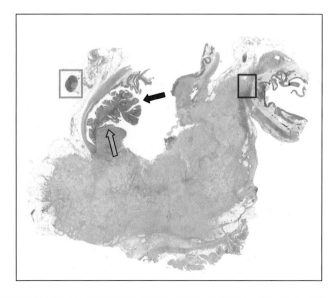

Fig. 3.**19 d**   Schematic guide to the morphologic details in the large section in Fig. 3.**19**.

# 4 Other Intestinal Neoplasms

## Case 4.1 Carcinoid Tumor of the Ileocecal Region

**Patient data:** 53-year-old man presenting with abdominal pain. Radiologic examination revealed stenosis of the terminal ileum.
**Surgical treatment:** Ileocecal resection, no preoperative treatment.
**Specimen:** 30-cm-long segment of the large intestine and an 8-cm part of the terminal ileum with a 5-cm infiltrating tumor mass with a yellow cut surface, in the area of the ileocecal valve.
**Histopathologic diagnosis:** Carcinoid tumor with lymph node metastasis (1/14).
**Follow-up:** Died of the disease 49 months after the operation.

The large section in Figure 4.1 demonstrates multiple round foci of tumor tissue invading all the layers of the wall of the small intestine. The section in fact corresponds to the ileocecal region and also contains structures of the colon (located in the left upper corner of the image). Microscopy revealed structures of carcinoid tumor corresponding to the red-colored areas in Figure 4.1 c. The tumor originated in the mucosa of the small intestine, as demonstrated in Figure 4.1 a, which is a microscopic magnification of the area marked with the yellow rectangle in the schematic image (Fig. 4.1 c). The tumor cells exhibited a strong immunohistochemical reaction with the endocrine marker chromogranin A (Fig. 4.1 b). Some lymph nodes free of metastasis were also present in the specimen (marked with green arrows in Fig. 4.1 c). The intestinal wall was thickened as a result of hypertrophy of the lamina muscularis propria, a typical phenomenon associated with carcinoid tumor. A deep ulceration is also seen at the distal end of the specimen.

### Practical points

- By including a transection of the entire tumor, large histologic sections provide an advantageous diagnostic tool in assessing the extent of tumor growth.
- Large sections allow examination of an extensive area of the mesocolon/mesenterium, which facilitates documenting locoregional metastatic tumor spread.

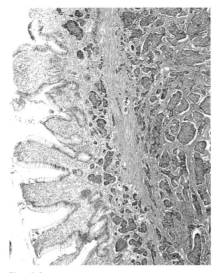

Fig. 4.1 a

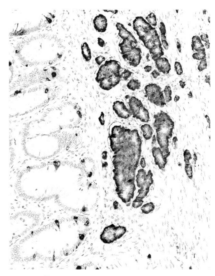

Fig. 4.1 b

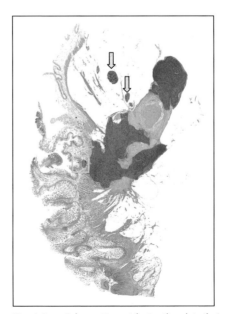

Fig. 4.1 c  Schematic guide to the details in the large section in Fig. 4.1.

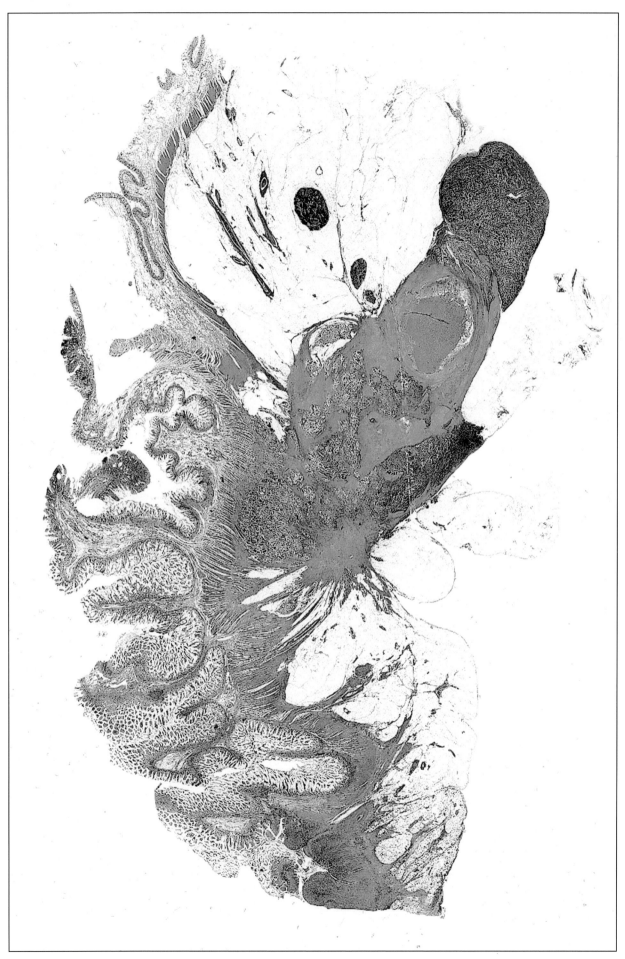

Fig. 4.**1**  Large-section histology image of carcinoid tumor of the ileocecal region.

## Case 4.2 Primary Malignant Lymphoma of the Colon

**Patient data:** 70-year-old-woman presenting with anemia. Colonoscopy revealed a large tumor mass in the cecum. The preoperative endoscopic biopsy contained mainly necrotic debris, thus raising suspicion of malignancy.

**Surgical treatment:** Ileocecal resection, no preoperative treatment.

**Specimen:** 50-cm-long segment of the large intestine together with an 8-cm part of the terminal ileum and tumorous appendix. A 10-cm infiltrating tumor was found in the cecum, and several tumor masses were found in the mesenterium.

**Histopathologic diagnosis:** Diffuse malignant non-Hodgkin's B-cell lymphoma of follicular origin, intermediate grade.

**Follow-up:** Died of the disease 7 months after the operation.

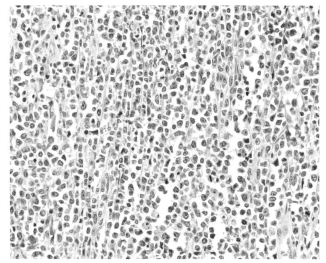

Fig. 4.**2 a**

The large histologic section in Figure 4.**2** demonstrates the typical appearance of a malignant lymphoma in the intestine: a diffuse, monotonous infiltrate leading to thickening of the intestinal wall due to discohesive growth of the tumor cells. The same monotonous histologic picture, seen in Figure 4.**2 a**, could be obtained by magnifying any part of the tumor. This lymphoma was made up of atypical B-lymphocytes (as shown by immunohistochemical reaction with the B-cell marker CD20, Fig. 4.**2 b**) and contained only a few reactive T-lymphocytes (Fig. 4.**2 c**, immunohistochemical reaction with CD3). The green arrow in Figure 4.**2 d** indicates the zone of transition between the normal intestinal structures and the tumor, the yellow arrow indicates areas of tumor necrosis. These areas may explain the results of the preoperative histologic examination in this case. Interestingly, there are reactive lymph nodes free of lymphoma in the immediate vicinity of the tumor (encircled in Fig. 4.**2 d**).

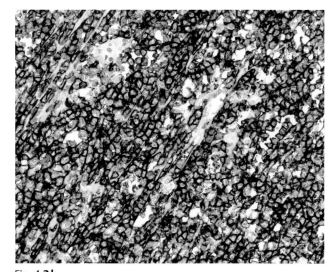

Fig. 4.**2 b**

### Practical points

- A diffuse solid thickening of the intestinal wall may indicate the presence of malignant lymphoma.
- Non-involved lymph nodes may be present in the immediate vicinity of a large mass of lymphoma, carrying the risk of a false-negative diagnosis when sampled for histologic examination.

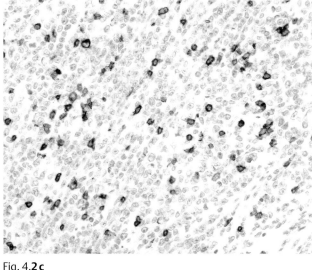

Fig. 4.**2 c**

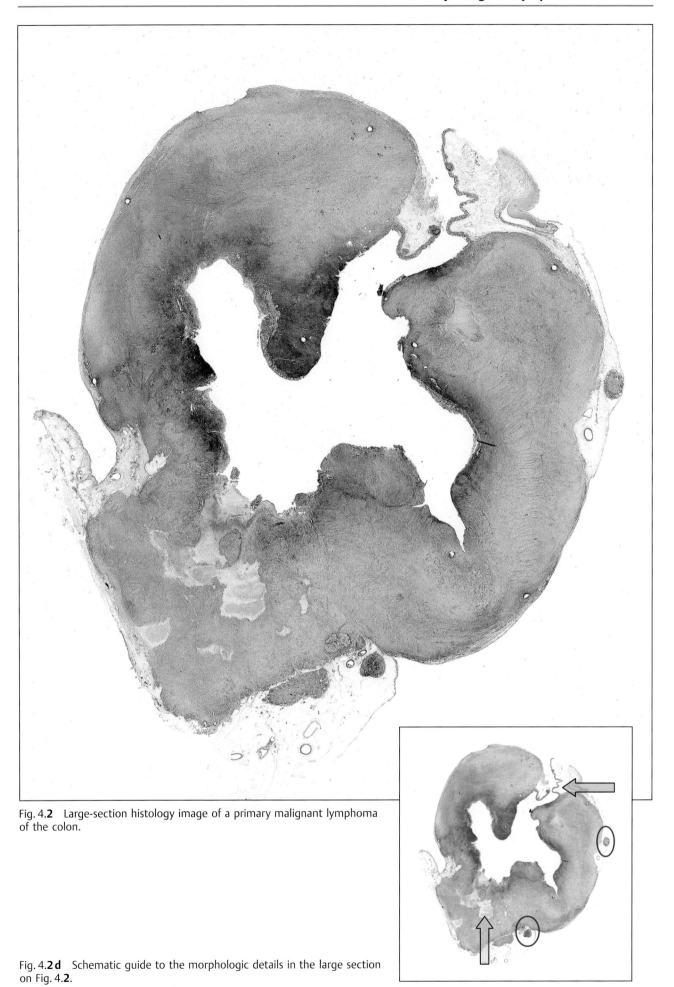

Fig. 4.2   Large-section histology image of a primary malignant lymphoma of the colon.

Fig. 4.2 d   Schematic guide to the morphologic details in the large section on Fig. 4.2.

## Case 4.3 Intestinal Lymphoma

**Patient data:** 88-year-old woman with previously diagnosed malignant lymphoma who presented with abdominal pain. On laparotomy, diffuse purulent peritonitis was detected and several independent tumor masses were seen in the small intestine. As a cause of peritonitis, intestinal perforation was found in one of the tumor-infiltrated segments.
**Surgical treatment:** Partial intestinal resection.
**Specimen:** 27-cm-long segment of the small intestine with a 6-cm-large tumor mass 3 cm from the margin. Additional smaller tumor masses were also present. Perforation in the area of the largest tumor and peritonitis.
**Histopathologic diagnosis:** Diffuse malignant non-Hodgkin's B-cell lymphoma of large-cell type, high-grade.
**Follow-up:** Died of the disease 12 months after the operation.

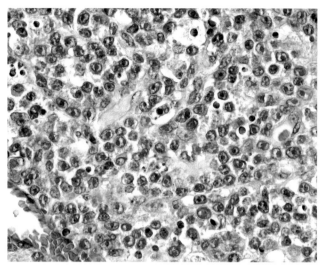

Fig. 4.**3 a**

The large histologic section in Figure 4.**3** demonstrates another case of malignant lymphoma, this time infiltrating the wall of the small intestine. The diffuse thickening of the intestinal wall is very well seen. As indicated by the yellow arrow in the schematic image (Fig. 4.**3 b**), the intestinal wall was perforated due to ulceration and necrosis of the tumor tissue. Necrotic areas were also present in other parts of the tumor; the most obvious of them is marked with a red rectangle in the schematic image. Figure 4.**3 a** is a microscopic magnification of a detail from the tissue of the high-grade lymphoma with large atypical cells containing prominent nucleoli.

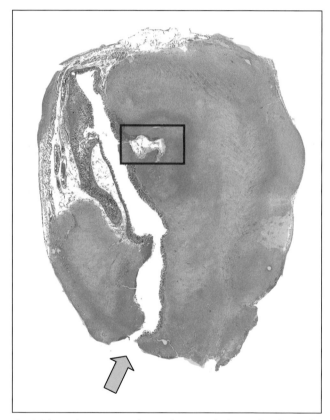

Fig. 4.**3 b**  Schematic guide to the morphologic details in the large section in Fig. 4.**3**.

**Practical points**

• Massive necrosis of malignant lymphoma tissues is frequent and may lead to perforation of the intestinal wall.

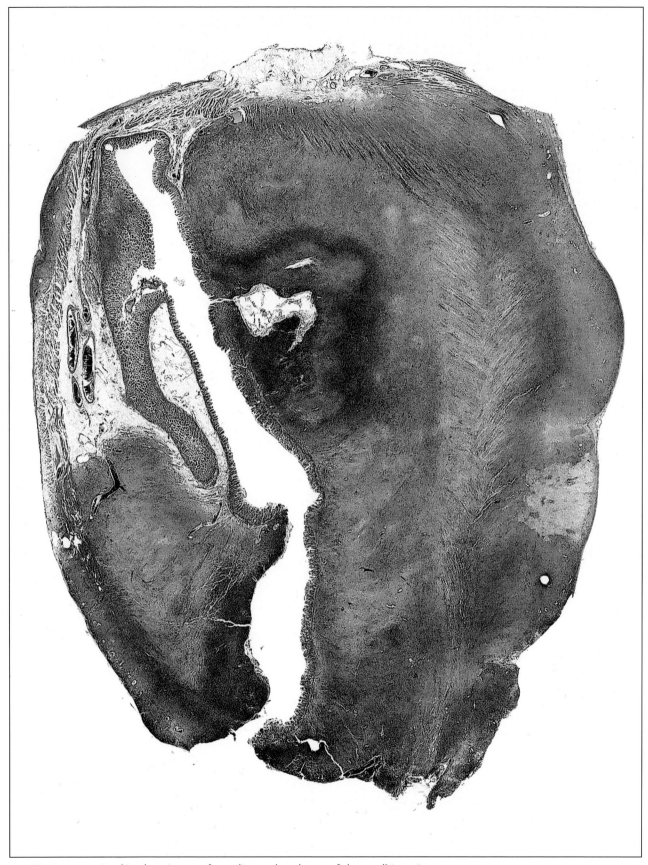

Fig. 4.**3**  Large-section histology image of a malignant lymphoma of the small intestine.

## Case 4.4 Intestinal Lymphoma with Massive Necrosis

**Patient data:** 61-year-old man presenting with episodes of abdominal pain. Colonoscopy revealed a large tumor mass in the cecum. Preoperative biopsy did not contain any tumor structures.
**Surgical treatment:** Right hemicolectomy, no preoperative treatment.
**Specimen:** Right hemicolectomy with 25-cm-long segment of the large intestine together with a 4-cm part of the terminal ileum and a 9-cm infiltrating tumor mass in the area of the ileocecal valve. Tumor mass in the mesenterium.
**Histopathologic diagnosis:** Diffuse malignant non-Hodgkin's B-cell lymphoma, intermediate grade.
**Follow-up:** 17 months, no signs of disease recurrence.

The large histologic section in Figure 4.**4** demonstrates a primary malignant lymphoma of the colon infiltrating the ileocecal region. The massive infiltration of the blue-stained tumor tissue is well seen in the mesenterium. There are large areas of tumor necrosis (indicated by the yellow-colored areas in Fig. 4.**4e**). The mucosa was only partly preserved and mostly ulcerated. Figure 4.**4a** is a microscopic magnification of the area indicated with the red rectangle in Figure 4.**4e** and demonstrates the intestinal mucosa on the right side of the image and the tissue of the lymphoma on the left side. Absence of a reaction with the epithelial marker cytokeratin Cam5,2 (illustrated in Fig. 4.**4b**) indicates a non-epithelial tumor (the rest of the normal epithelium is stained brown). Figure 4.**4c, d** is a high-power microscopic magnification of the lymphoma and also proves the aggressive nature of the tumor, which shows perivascular and intramuscular infiltration. Note the enlarged reactive lymph node (marked with a blue arrow in Fig. 4.**4e**). Massive necrosis of the tumor tissue may appear in lymphomas as well as in carcinomas and can lead to the formation of pseudolumen, as was already demonstrated in Case 3.14.

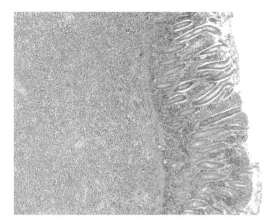

Fig. 4.**4a**

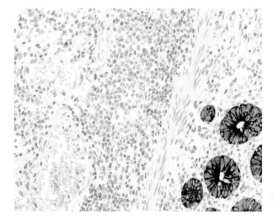

Fig. 4.**4b**

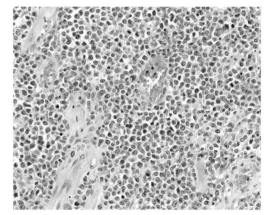

Fig. 4.**4c**

**Practical points**

- Massive necrosis of the tissue of malignant lymphomas is frequent and may lead to perforation of the intestinal wall or to formation of a pseudolumen.

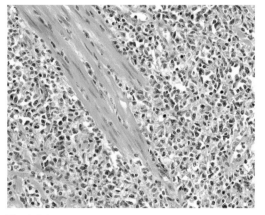

Fig. 4.**4d**

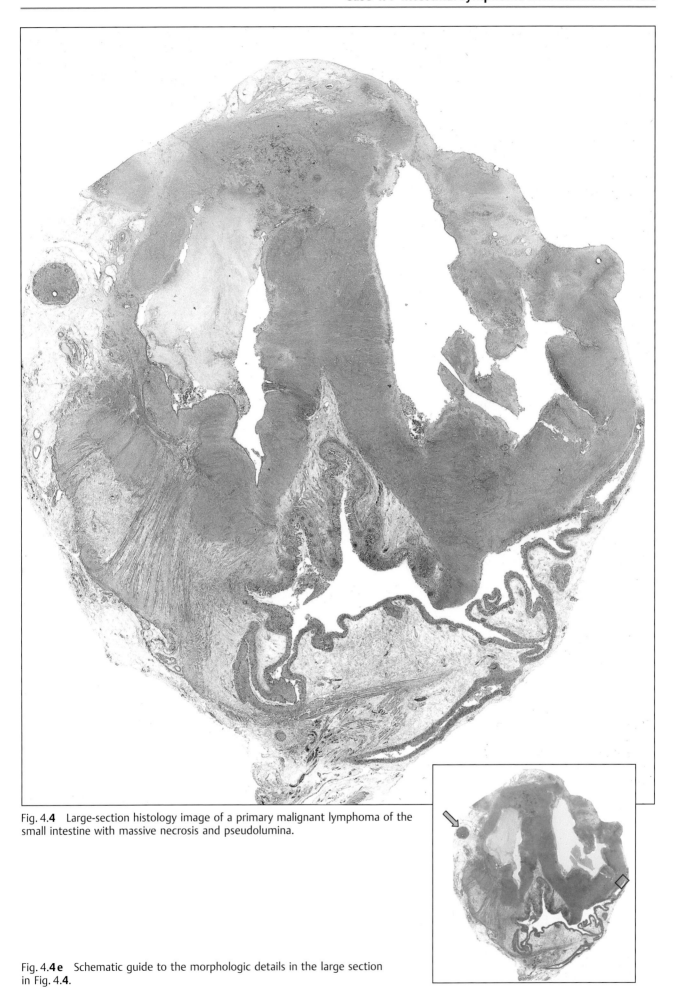

Fig. 4.**4**  Large-section histology image of a primary malignant lymphoma of the small intestine with massive necrosis and pseudolumina.

Fig. 4.**4e**  Schematic guide to the morphologic details in the large section in Fig. 4.**4**.

## Case 4.5 Intestinal Lymphoma Presenting as Polyposis

**Patient data:** 68-year-old man presenting with acute abdominal pain. Invagination of a segment in the jejunum was seen on laparotomy.
**Surgical treatment:** Partial resection of the jejunum, no preoperative treatment.
**Specimen:** 75-cm-long segment of the small intestine showing hemorrhagic infarction in the central part. A large number of polypoid tumors, measuring 1–25 mm, were seen in the mucosal surface of the intestine.
**Histopathologic diagnosis:** Multiple lymphomatous polyps of the small intestine (malignant intestinal non-Hodgkin's B-cell lymphoma, mantle-zone lymphoma); hemorrhagic infarction.
**Follow-up:** 4 months, no signs of disease recurrence.

Another typical appearance of intestinal lymphoma is polyposis. As demonstrated in the large histologic section in Figure 4.**5**, the tumor may form several independent nodules in the submucosa, bulging out from the mucosal surface as polyps. The larger tumor masses may become ulcerated. The individual tumor foci are marked with yellow arrows in the schematic image (Fig. 4.**5 e**). Four small tumor foci are microscopically magnified in Figure 4.**5 a**. Figure 4.**5 b** represents a histologic detail of the lymphoma. Two immunohistochemical images are also presented: (1) cytokeratin Cam 5,2 demonstrating the epithelial structures in the mucosa and leaving the lymphoma cells (left upper part of the image) unstained (Fig. 4.**5 c**), and (2) bcl-2, staining the cells of the lymphoma and leaving the epithelium unstained (Fig. 4.**5 d**).

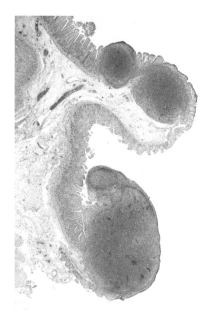

Fig. 4.**5 a**

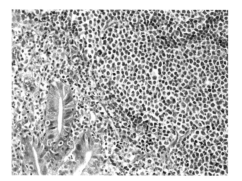

Fig. 4.**5 b**

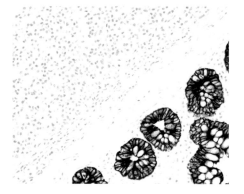

Fig. 4.**5 c**

**Practical points**

- Some malignant lymphomas may present as multiple polyps in the lumen of the intestine.
- The large histologic section, by including several polypoid lesions together with their environment, aids in making the proper diagnosis.

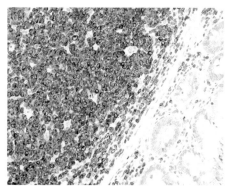

Fig. 4.**5 d**

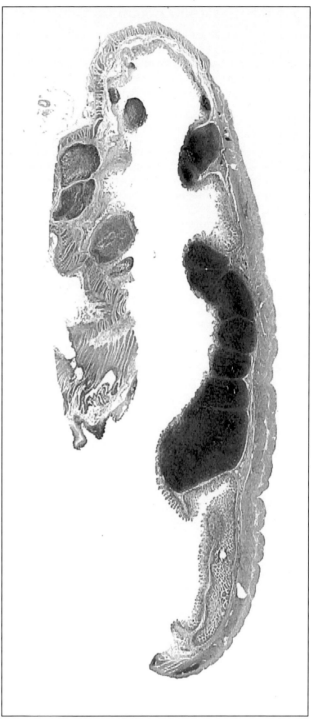

Fig. 4.**5**   Large-section histology image of a primary malignant lymphoma of the small intestine presenting as polyposis.

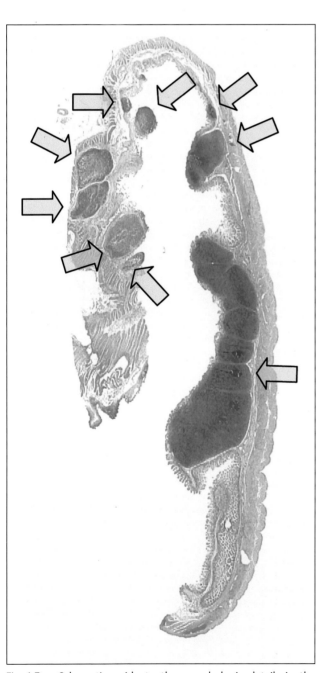

Fig. 4.**5 e**   Schematic guide to the morphologic details in the large section in Fig. 4.**5**.

## Case 4.6 Gastrointestinal Stromal Tumor

**Patient data:** 51-year-old man presenting with episodic abdominal pain. Computer tomography revealed an abdominal tumor in connection with a loop of the small intestine.

**Surgical treatment:** Partial resection of the jejunum, no preoperative treatment.

**Specimen:** 20-cm-long segment of the small intestine centrally with a 7 × 5-cm circumscribed tumor with a small ulceration on the mucosal surface.

**Histopathologic diagnosis:** Gastrointestinal stromal tumor (GIST) of the small intestine.

**Follow-up:** 34 months, no signs of disease recurrence.

This large histologic section demonstrates the typical appearance of GIST in the small intestine (Fig. 4.**6**). The tumor is egg-shaped, with an „umbilication" located centrally in the part of the mucosa, which covers the tumor. The area of the tumor is green-colored in the schematic image (Fig. 4.**6 d**). The „umbilication" often seen endoscopically in these cases represents ulceration, typically appearing in the central portion of the part of the mucosa covering the GIST. This ulceration, corresponding to the area of the red rectangle in Figure 4.**6 d**, is magnified in Figure 4.**6 a**. The tumor consisted of relatively monomorphous spindle cells (as demonstrated in the histologic image, Fig. 4.**6 b**) and showed a strong immunohistochemical reaction to CD117, a marker regularly expressed by GISTs (Fig. 4.**6 c**).

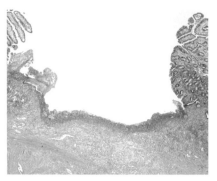

Fig. 4.**6 a**

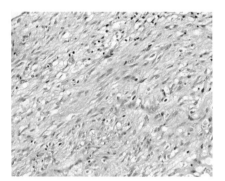

Fig. 4.**6 b**

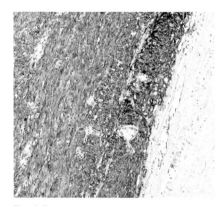

Fig. 4.**6 c**

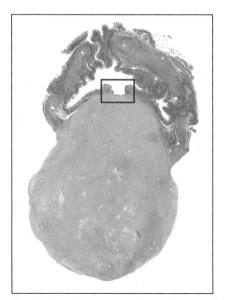

Fig. 4.**6 d**  Schematic guide to the morphologic details in the large section in Fig. 4.**6**.

### Practical points

- In cases of GIST, as in other tumors, large histologic sections may include a transection of the entire tumor together with the intestinal wall, which allows diagnosis, typing and grading of the lesion to be done at the same time.
- The growth pattern of GIST, as demonstrated in large sections, is typical and different from those of carcinomas and lymphomas.

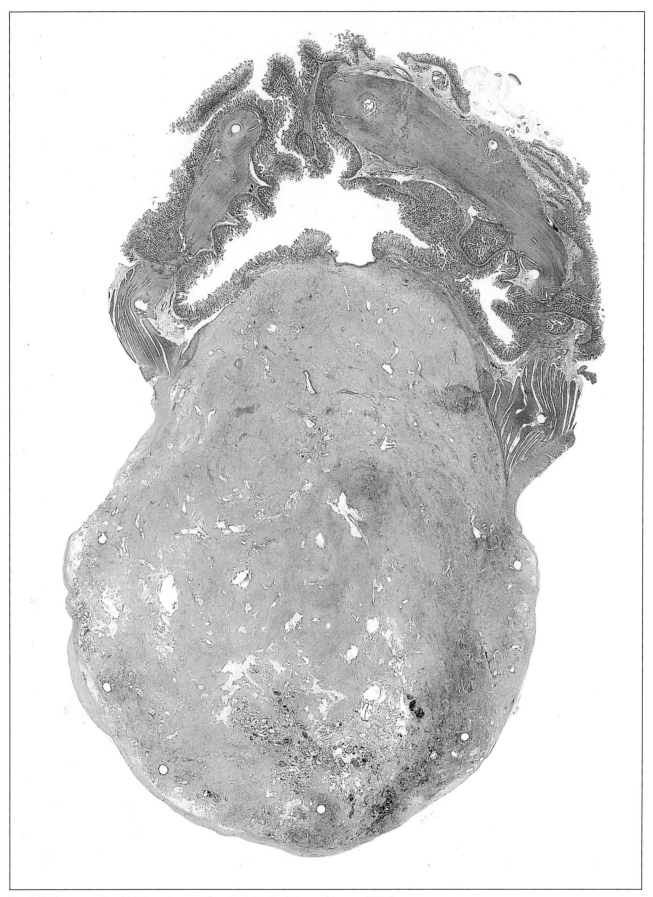

Fig. 4.6  Large-section histology image of gastrointestinal stromal tumor (GIST).

## Case 4.7 Gastrointestinal Stromal Tumor

**Patient data:** 65-year-old woman who underwent surgery for a suspicious ovarian tumor. During the operation, a large tumor mass was detected in her jejunum.
**Surgical treatment:** Partial resection of the jejunum, no preoperative treatment.
**Specimen:** 8-cm-long segment of the small intestine centrally with a 4.5 cm well circumscribed tumor mass.
**Histopathologic diagnosis:** GIST of the small intestine. Simple cyst in the right ovary.
**Follow-up:** 32 months, no signs of disease recurrence.

Figure 4.7 demonstrates a large histologic section of another case of GIST. The area of the tumor tissue is green-colored in the schematic image (Fig. 4.7d). The sandglass-like shape of the tumor is very well seen. In this particular case, the neoplasm elevated and attenuated the overlying mucosa. On histologic examination, the tumor exhibited a storiform pattern of growth (Fig. 4.7a) and focally obvious cellular atypia (Fig. 4.7b). Furthermore, as a consequence of tumor necrosis, large "empty" spaces are seen in the tumor, partly filled with blood. These spaces are marked with the red arrows in the schematic image and one of them is partially presented magnified in Figure 4.7c.

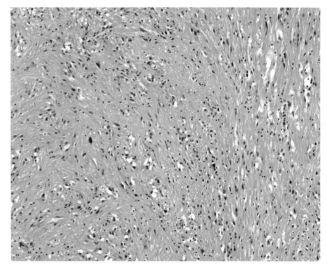
Fig. 4.7a

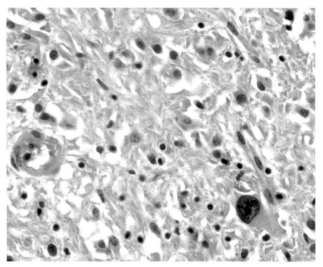
Fig. 4.7b

**Practical points**

- Larger solid tumors often exhibit "empty" spaces of different size on large section histology as a consequence of tumor necrosis.

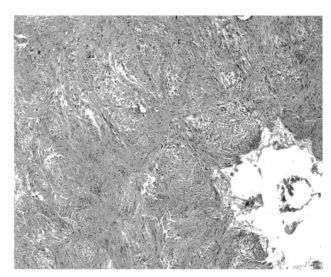
Fig. 4.7c

Fig. 4.**7d**   Schematic guide to the morphologic details in the large section in Fig. 4.**7**.

Fig. 4.**7**   Large-section histology image of a gastrointestinal stromal tumor (GIST).

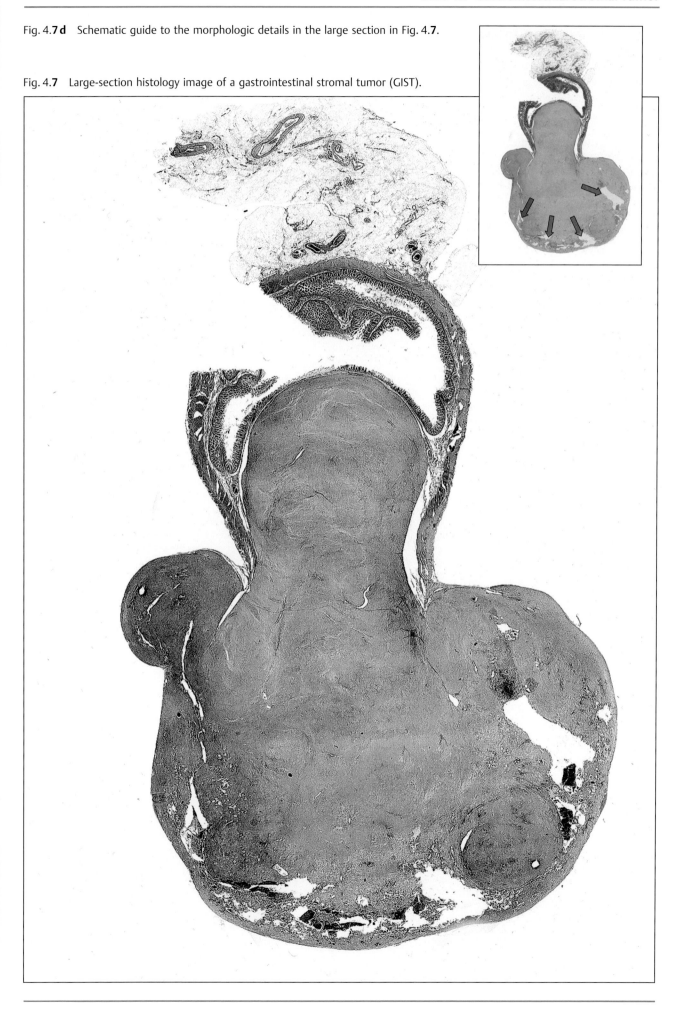

## Case 4.8 Gastrointestinal Stromal Tumor

**Patient data:** 61-year-old woman presenting with intermittent abdominal pain and severe anemia. Endoscopically, a large submucosal tumor was seen in the colon ascendens.

**Surgical treatment:** Right hemicolectomy, no preoperative treatment.

**Specimen:** Right hemicolectomy with 22-cm-long segment of the large intestine, 8-cm-long part of the terminal ileum and a 9-cm well circumscribed tumor mass in the wall of the colon.

**Histopathologic diagnosis:** GIST of the large intestine.

**Follow-up:** 2 months, no signs of disease recurrence.

The large histologic section in Figure **4.8** demonstrates a GIST growing in the wall of the large intestine. The area of the tumor tissue is green-colored in the schematic image (Fig. **4.8c**). The specimen was received open; thus the mucosa is seen along the left side of the tumor. The tumor was sharply delineated towards the mucosa, which remained intact, as demonstrated magnified in Figure **4.8a**, (the corresponding area is marked with the red rectangle in the schematic image, Fig. **4.8c**). In this particular case, the neoplasm is lobulated and shows obvious intratumoral heterogeneity. The main part of the tumor exhibits the typical histologic picture of a GIST, with storiform structures and somewhat atypical tumor cells (Fig. **4.8b**). There were also paucicellular fibrotic areas with microcalcifications (indicated with yellow arrows in Fig. **4.8c**). Note also the two reactive lymph nodes, indicated with orange arrows in the schematic image.

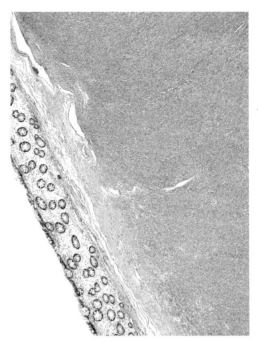

Fig. 4.**8a**

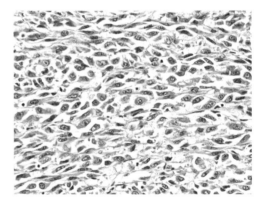

Fig. 4.**8b**

### Practical points

- By including a transsection of the whole solid tumor, the large histologic sections facilitate the demonstration of intratumoral heterogeneity.

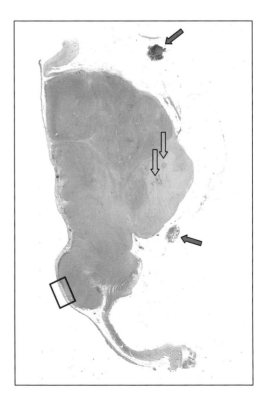

Fig. 4.**8c** Schematic guide to the morphologic details in the large section on Fig. **4.8**.

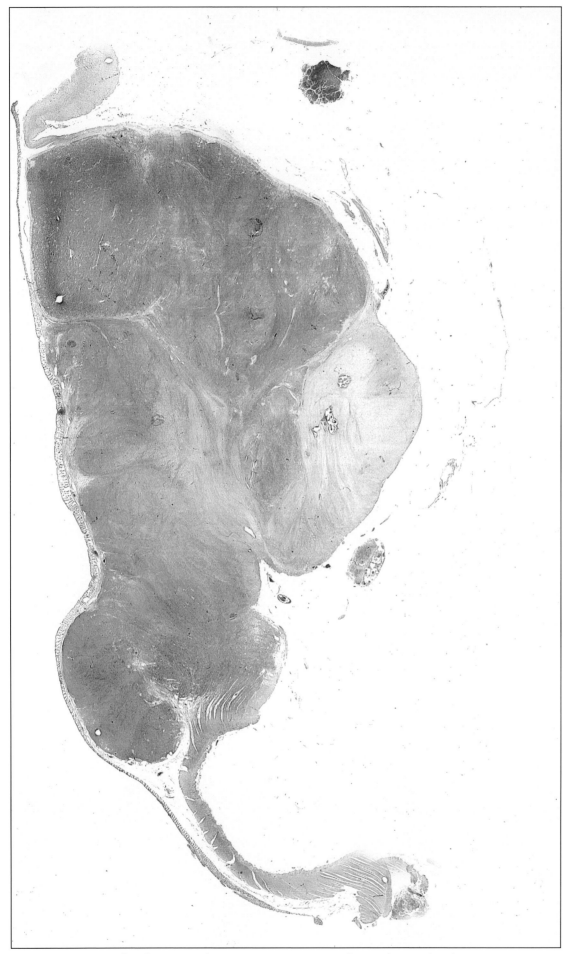

Fig. 4.**8** Large-section histology image demonstrating gastrointestinal stromal tumor (GIST).

## Case 4.9 Submucosal Lipoma

**Patient data:** 45-year-old man presenting with bloody diarrhea. Endoscopically, a round broad-based tumor-like structure was seen in the descendent colon. Repeated biopsies revealed only signs consistent with a chronic inflammatory process. The patient underwent surgery based on clinical indications.

**Surgical treatment:** Left hemicolectomy, no preoperative treatment.

**Specimen:** 18-cm-long segment of the large intestine centrally with a 4 × 3-cm submucosal lipoma.

**Histopathologic diagnosis:** Submucosal lipoma of the colon, no signs of malignancy.

**Follow-up:** 18 months, no signs of disease recurrence.

The large-section image (Fig. 4.**9**) demonstrates a submucosal tumor, consisting of mature fatty tissue. The tumor corresponds to the yellow-colored area in the schematic image (Fig. 4.**9d**). The mucosa contained irregular and hyperplastic crypts without signs of active inflammatory reaction, as demonstrated in Figure 4.**9a**, which is a microscopic magnification of the area marked with the blue rectangle in the schematic image. Centrally, over the tumor, the mucosa is ulcerated (Fig. 4.**9b**, corresponding to the area of the red rectangle in Fig. 4.**9d**). Figure 4.**9c** is a magnified image of a detail from the lipoma. A reactive lymph node, marked with the green arrow in the schematic image, is also present in the specimen.

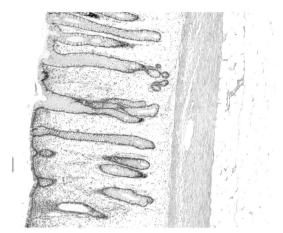

Fig. 4.**9a**

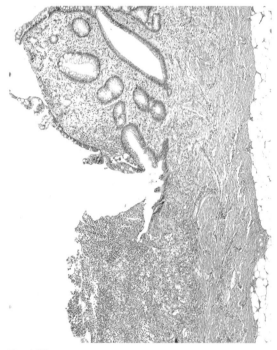

Fig. 4.**9b**

**Practical points**

- Like other neoplasias, lipomas may be reliably documented using large histologic sections. Their location, frequently in the submucosa, is easily seen. The growth pattern of a lipoma is different from those of carcinomas or lymphomas.

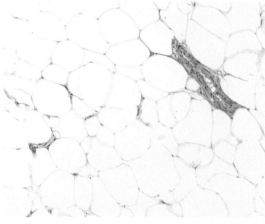

Fig. 4.**9c**

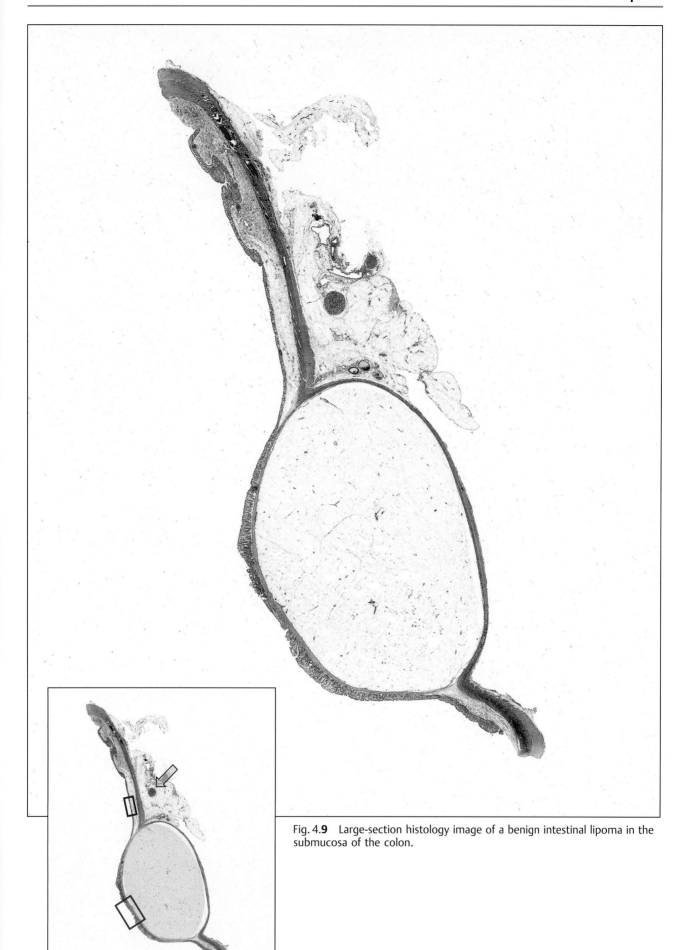

Fig. 4.**9**  Large-section histology image of a benign intestinal lipoma in the submucosa of the colon.

Fig. 4.**9 d**  Schematic guide to the morphologic details in the large section in Fig. 4.**9**.

# 5 Non-neoplastic Lesions

## Case 5.1 Ulcerative Colitis

**Patient data:** 66-year-old man with a 15-year history of ulcerative colitis, currently non-responding to therapy.
**Surgical treatment:** Colectomy, after long-term medication for the disease.
**Specimen:** 120-cm-long large intestine together with a 4-cm part of the terminal ileum. Ulcerations in the distal part of the specimen. No polyps or tumors.
**Histopathologic diagnosis:** Active ulcerative colitis. No dysplasia. No malignancy.
**Follow-up:** 16 months, no signs of recurrence of the disease.

The large section in Figure 5.**1** demonstrates the typical morphological appearance of ulcerative colitis. The main pathological changes in this disease are restricted to the mucosa. The submucosa shows only signs of edema; larger numbers of inflammatory cells are not seen. The lamina muscularis propria is intact. In the schematic image (Fig. 5.**1 d**), the mucosa is indicated with a red arrowhead, the submucosa with a yellow one and the lamina muscularis propria with a green one. Figure 5.**1 a** represents a low-power magnification of the bowel wall, including all the indicated layers, in the area of the yellow rectangle in the schematic image. The magnified detail in Figure 5.**1 b** demonstrates the edematous submucosa, which is free of inflammatory cells. The distortion of the crypts is also well seen. Figure 5.**1 c** is a detail from the mucosa, illustrating intensive active inflammation with a collection of granulocytes in the lumen of a distorted gland (so-called cryptal abscess). Several lymph nodes are also present in the specimen (marked with the green arrows in the schematic image, Fig. 5.**1 d**).

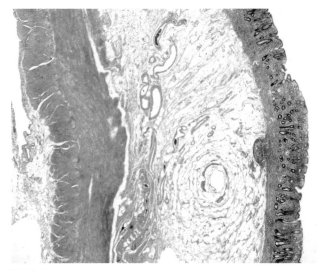

Fig. 5.**1 a**

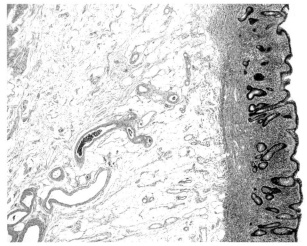

Fig. 5.**1 b**

**Practical points**

- Inclusion of an entire transection of the intestine in a single large histologic section is advantageous not only with respect to tumor pathology, but also when assessing the extent and distribution of inflammatory lesions.
- Inflammation mostly restricted to the mucosa is typical of ulcerative colitis.

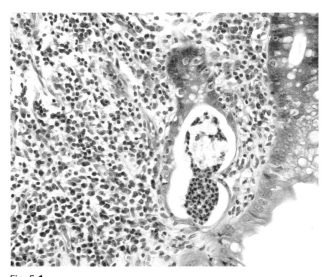

Fig. 5.**1 c**

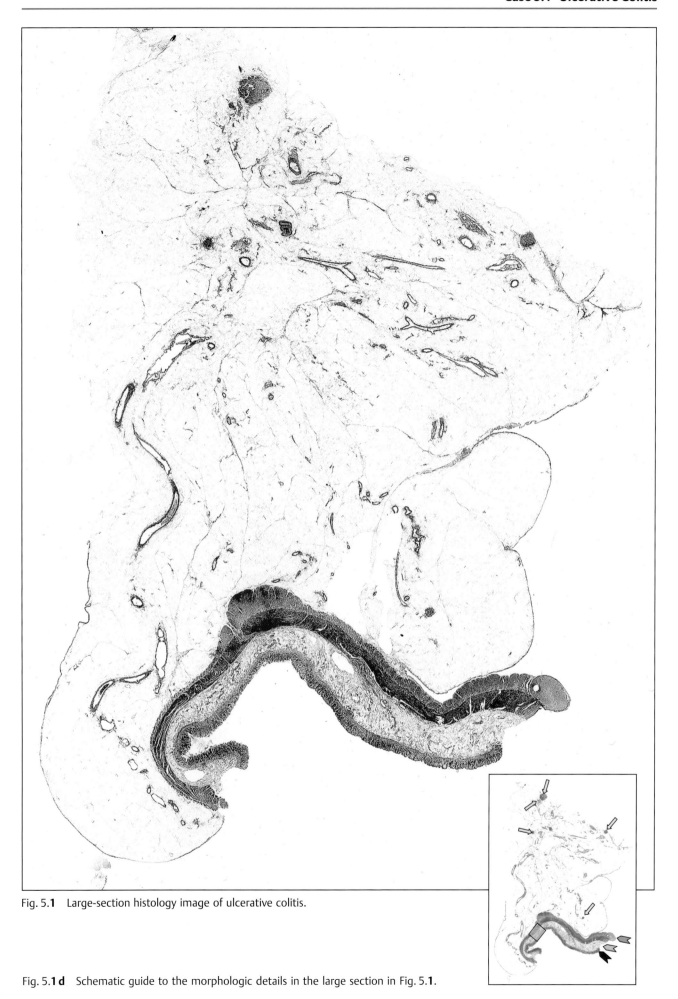

Fig. 5.**1**   Large-section histology image of ulcerative colitis.

Fig. 5.**1 d**   Schematic guide to the morphologic details in the large section in Fig. 5.**1**.

## Case 5.2 Crohn's Disease

**Patient data:** 53-year-old man with a long history of Crohn's disease, presenting with abdominal pain. Previously operated on for intestinal obstruction caused by Crohn's disease.

**Surgical treatment:** Ileocecal resection.

**Specimen:** 15-cm-long segment of the large intestine together with an 8-cm part of the terminal ileum and 4-cm appendix. The walls of the terminal ileum and proximal part of the cecum were thickened, the lumen narrowed, and the mucosa partly ulcerated.

**Histopathologic diagnosis:** Crohn's disease of the terminal ileum and cecum. No signs of malignancy.

**Follow-up:** 1 month, no signs of disease recurrence.

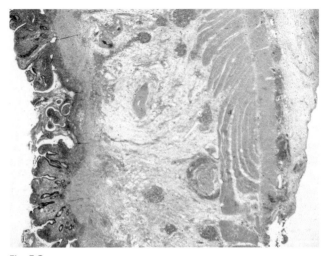

Fig. 5.**2a**

Although somewhat tangentially sectioned, the large histologic section in Figure 5.**2** reliably demonstrates the hallmark of Crohn's disease: transmural inflammation leading to thickening of the intestinal wall. Figure 5.**2a** represents a low-power magnification of the area corresponding to the yellow rectangle in the schematic image (Fig. 5.**2d**) and illustrates the presence of inflammatory changes in all layers of the intestinal wall. Deep mucosal ulcerations are seen as well as the lymphoid follicles in the submucosa and subserosa. The submucosa is edematous, thickened (as indicated with the blue double-arrow in the schematic image) and contains inflammatory cells. A deep ulceration with incipient fissure formation is demonstrated in Figure 5.**2b** (corresponding to the area of the red rectangle in Fig. 5.**2d**). Comparison with the previous large-section image (Case 5.1) clearly shows the differences between ulcerative colitis and Crohn's disease. As a hallmark of Crohn's disease, epithelioid granulomas were found in the intestinal wall and in the lymph nodes. A lymph node containing granulomas (indicated with the blue arrow in the schematic image) is microscopically magnified in Figure 5.**2c**.

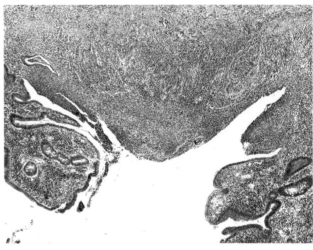

Fig. 5.**2b**

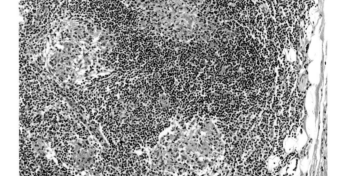

### Practical points

- Transmural inflammation, the hallmark of Crohn's disease, even when only focal, is easily seen in large sections.

Fig. 5.**2c**

Fig. 5.**2 d**   Schematic guide to the details in the large section in Fig. 5.**2**.

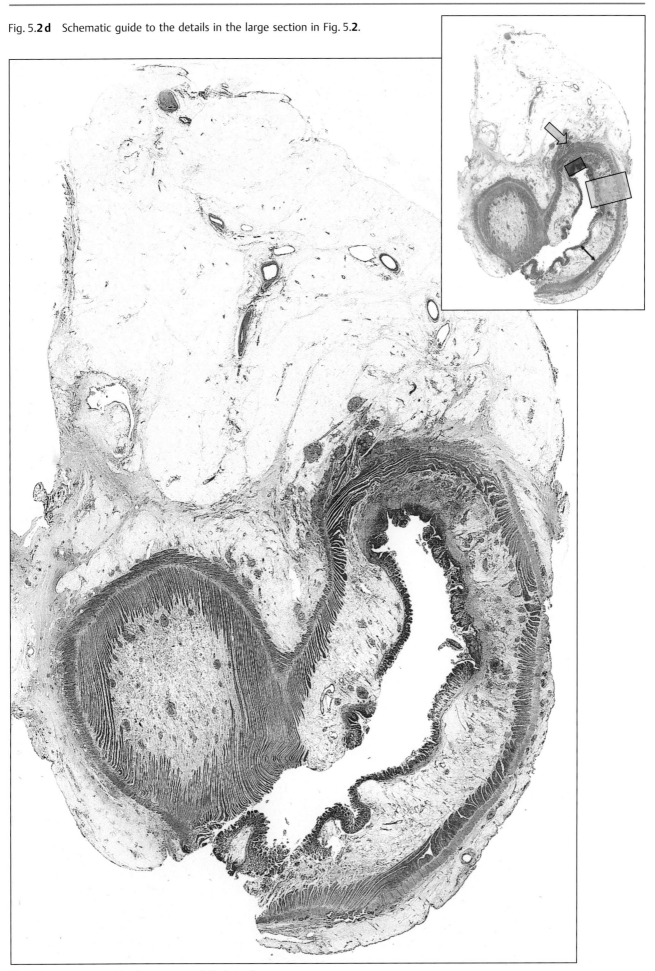

Fig. 5.**2** Large-section histology image of Crohn's disease.

## Case 5.3 Crohn's Disease

**Patient data:** 46-year-old woman presenting with abdominal pain. Radiologic examination revealed stenosis of the terminal ileum.
**Surgical treatment:** Ileocecal resection, no preoperative treatment.
**Specimen:** 10-cm-long segment of the large intestine together with an 18-cm part of the terminal ileum, with a thickened wall, pseudopolyps, and ulcerations on the mucosal surface.
**Histopathologic diagnosis:** Crohn's disease in the terminal ileum.
**Follow-up:** 8 months, no signs of disease recurrence.

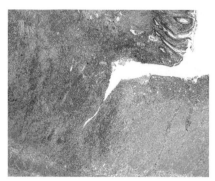

Fig. 5.**3a**

This large histologic section in Figure 5.**3** demonstrates another case of Crohn's disease. Pseudopolyps, wide ulcerations, transmural inflammation, and a pericolic abscess are seen. The pseudopolyps are indicated with yellow arrows in the schematic image (Fig. 5.**3e**). The blue rectangle in the schematic image indicates a fissure, magnified microscopically in Figure 5.**3a**. Figure 5.**3b** illustrates a deep ulceration and part of a pseudopolyp (corresponding to the red-colored area in Fig. 5.**3e**). An undermining ulceration is present in the blue-colored area in the schematic image and is histologically magnified in Figure 5.**3c**. The pericolic abscess marked with a yellow rectangle in Figure 5.**3s** is seen magnified in Figure 5.**3d**. Compared to the previous case (Case 5.2), the present image illustrates a more advanced stage of Crohn's disease.

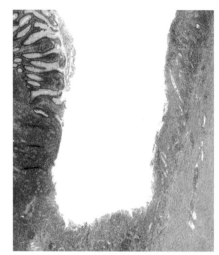

Fig. 5.**3b**

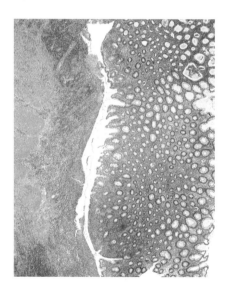

Fig. 5.**3c**

### Practical points

- Inclusion of an entire transection of the intestine into a single large histologic section is advantageous not only with respect to tumor pathology, but also when assessing the extent and distribution of inflammatory lesions.
- Large, non-fragmented histologic images assist in making the proper differential diagnosis of the subtypes of inflammatory bowel disease.

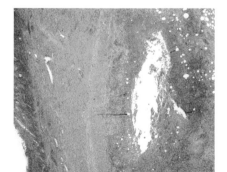

Fig. 5.**3d**

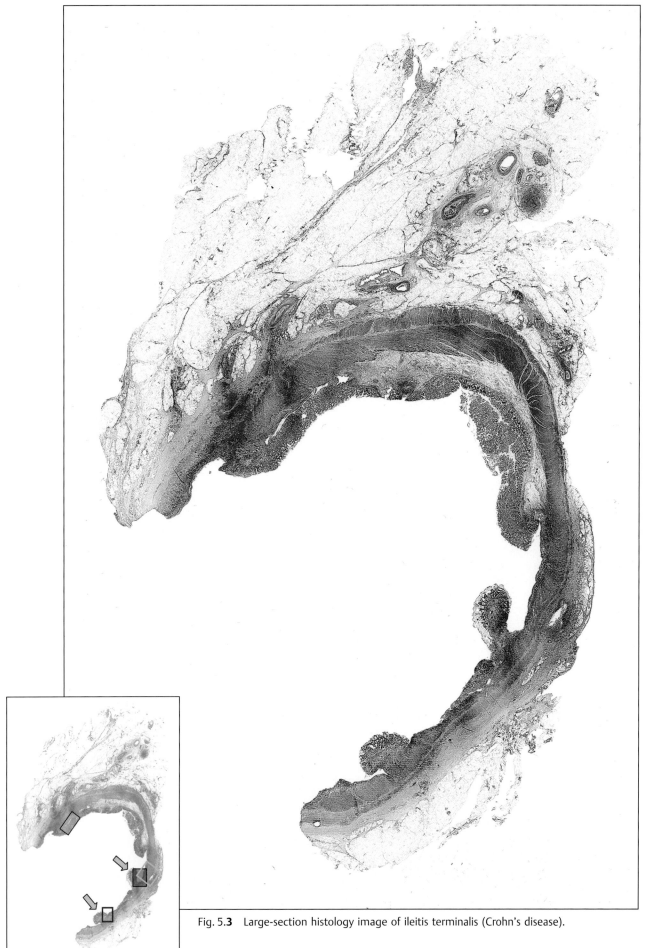

Fig. 5.**3**    Large-section histology image of ileitis terminalis (Crohn's disease).

Fig. 5.**3 e**    Schematic guide to the morphologic details in the large section in Fig. 5.**3**.

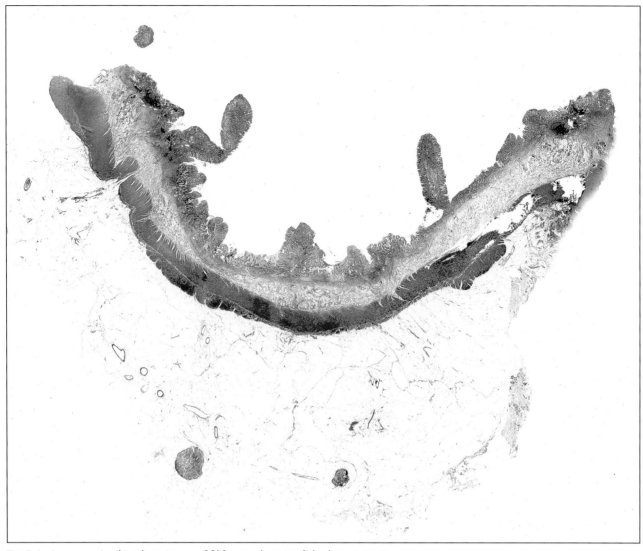

Fig. 5.**4**  Large-section histology image of filiform polyposis of the large intestine.

## Case 5.4 Filiform Polyposis of the Large Intestine

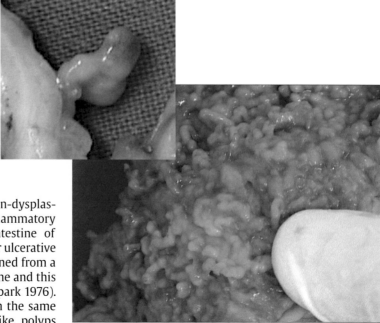

Multiple leaf-like polyps covered by normal (non-dysplastic and non-hyperplastic, but often showing inflammatory changes) mucosa may be present in the intestine of patients with a long history of Crohn's disease or ulcerative colitis. The large section in Figure 5.**4** was obtained from a patient with Crohn's disease of the large intestine and this condition, which is called filiform polyposis. (Spark 1976). Figure 5.**4a** is a macroscopic image taken from the same patient and shows hundreds of small leaf-like polyps covering the intestinal mucosa.

Fig. 5.**4a**

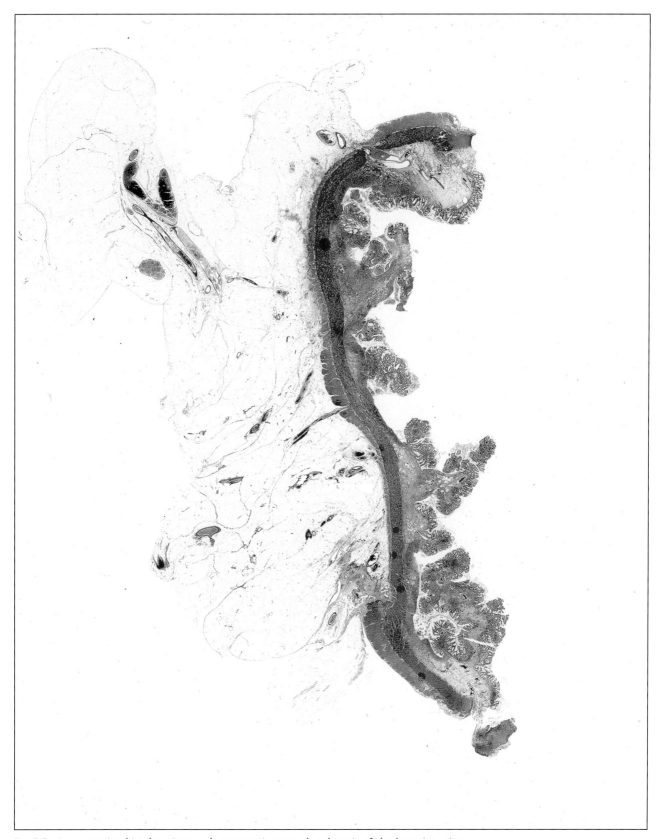

Fig. 5.**5**   Large-section histology image demonstrating pseudopolyposis of the large intestine.

## Case 5.5 Pseudopolyps of the Large Intestine in Ulcerative Colitis

This large histologic section in Figure 5.**5** demonstrates a transection of the large intestine with signs of chronic ulcerative colitis. As a consequence of deep and wide ulceration and protrusion of the mucosa, polyp-like structures have formed. The intestinal wall is of normal thickness and the pathological process is limited to the mucosa and to the submucosa. Compared to the previous two cases (Cases 5.3 and 5.4), the findings are similar but more superficial.

## Case 5.6 Closed Rectal Stump with Severe Inflammatory Changes

**Patient data:** 62-year-old man with ileostomy and closed rectal stump, presenting with rectal pain and bleeding. The patient underwent colectomy on indication of therapy-resistant ulcerative colitis 8 years before the present operation.

**Surgical treatment:** Resection of the rectal stump, no preoperative irradiation.

**Specimen:** 12-cm-long rectum with deep mucosal ulcerations and fibrosis.

**Histopathologic diagnosis:** Inflammatory lesions corresponding to ulcerative proctitis in a rectal stump. Three reactive lymph nodes. No malignancy.

**Follow-up:** 18 months, no signs of disease recurrence.

This patient underwent colectomy because of therapy-resistant ulcerative colitis 8 years before the present operation. He had an ileostomy and a preserved closed rectal stump. Moderate to severe inflammatory changes in the rectal stump are common in this situation (Winther et al. 2004). A transection of the resected rectum is demonstrated in the large section in Figure 5.**6**. The deep mucosal ulcerations causing bleeding and inflammation are well seen. Two histologic details are microscopically magnified in Figure 5.**6a**, **b** (corresponding to the orange- and yellow-colored areas, respectively, in the schematic image, Fig. 5.**6c**) in order to further illustrate the process. The large section also shows an enlarged reactive lymph node (marked with the green arrow in the schematic image).

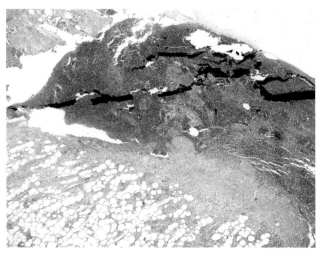

Fig. 5.**6a**

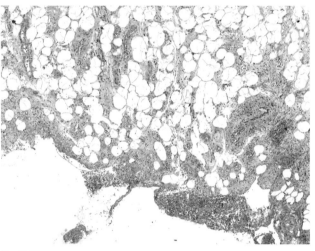

Fig. 5.**6b**

### Practical points

- Including a contiguous piece of tissue several centimeters in size in a single histologic section is also advantageous when studying infrequently diagnosed, unusual intestinal lesions.

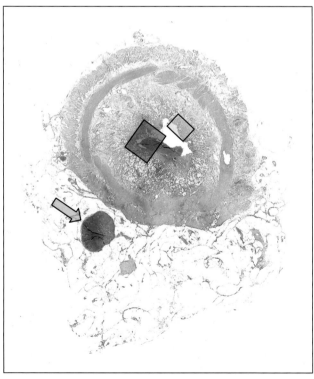

Fig. 5.**6c** Schematic guide to the morphologic details in the large section in Fig. 5.**6**.

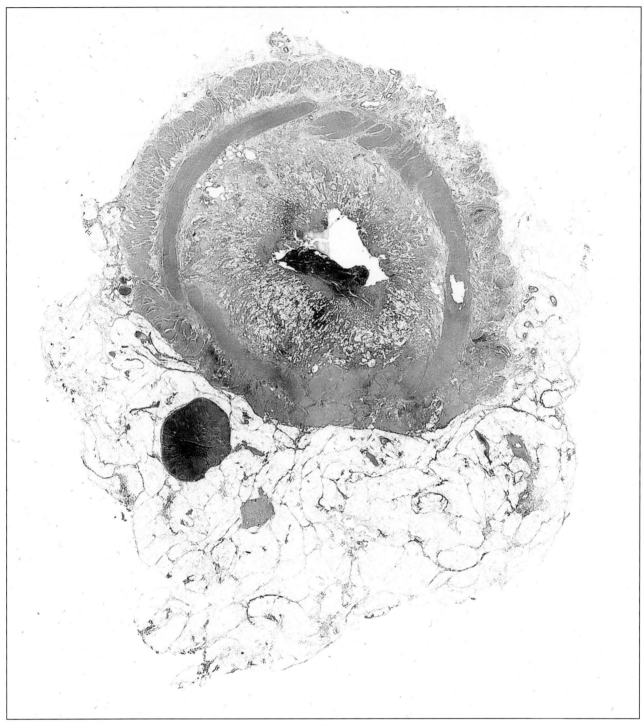

Fig. 5.**6** Large-section histology image of a rectal stump with inflammatory changes.

## Case 5.7 Diverticulosis of the Colon

**Patient data:** 57-year-old man presenting with a long history of recurrent abdominal pain.
**Surgical treatment:** Sigmoidal resection, no preoperative treatment.
**Specimen:** 15-cm-long segment of the large intestine; macroscopically, with multiple diverticles and focal peridiverticular inflammation.
**Histopathologic diagnosis:** Diverticulosis coli, diverticulitis and peridiverticular inflammation. No malignancy.
**Follow-up:** 87 months, no signs of disease recurrence.

Diverticulosis of the colon is a frequent pathologic condition. It is often associated with an inflammatory reaction and sometimes leads to the formation of tumor-like masses. The large histologic section in Figure 5.**7** demonstrates not only multiple diverticles in the same section plane (marked with the yellow arrows in the schematic image, Fig. 5.**7 b**) but also the pseudopolypoid appearance of the interdiverticular mucosa. The lamina muscularis propria is hyperplastic. There are two lymph nodes in the section (marked with red circles in the schematic image). In this patient, the symptoms of the disease were recurrent and related to inflammation around some of the diverticles. This inflammation may involve also the peritoneum locally, as is illustrated in this particular case. The area corresponding to the blue rectangle in Figure 5.**7 b** shows an intensive active inflammatory infiltrate with neutrophil granulocytes present. A microscopic detail from this area is seen magnified in Figure 5.**7 a**.

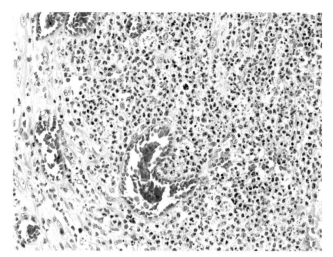

Fig. 5.**7 a**

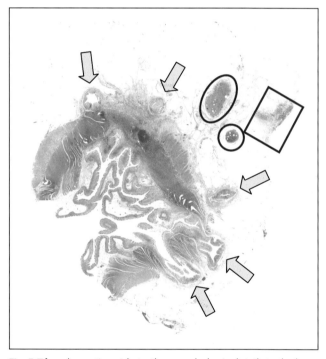

Fig. 5.**7 b**  chematic guide to the morphologic details in the large section in Fig. 5.**7**.

**Practical points**

- Inclusion into a single section of an entire transection of the large intestine together with its surrounding tissue gives a non-fragmented image properly demonstrating multiple lesions and their relation to each other.

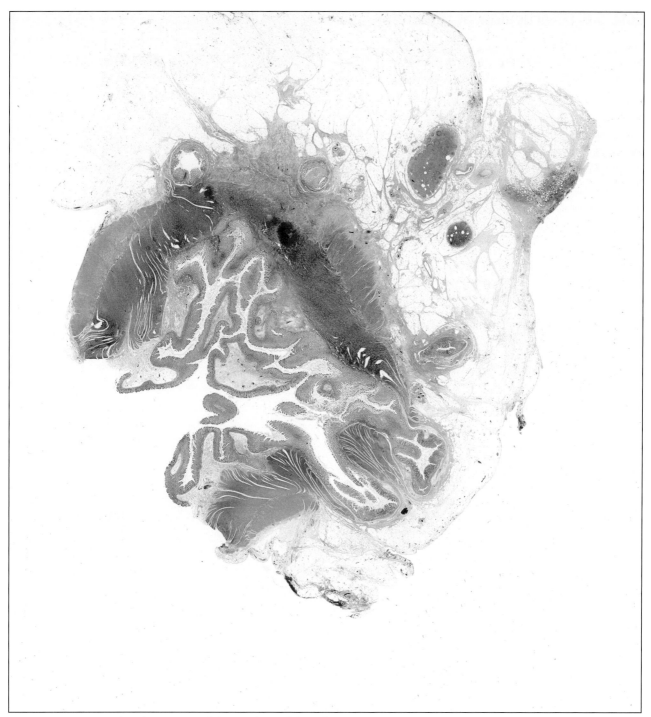

Fig. 5.**7**   Large-section histology image of diverticulosis of the colon.

## Case 5.8 Diverticulitis of the Colon

**Patient data:** 71-year-old man presenting with signs of acute intestinal obstruction. During laparotomy, a tumor-like lesion was seen in the sigmoid colon, which was adherent to the surrounding structures, indicating a need for partial resection of the urinary bladder and ureter.
**Surgical treatment:** Sigmoidal resection together with adherent structures, no preoperative treatment.
**Specimen:** 16-cm-long segment of the large intestine together with an adherent part of the urinary bladder and ureter.
**Histopathologic diagnosis:** Diverticulosis coli. Peridiverticular abscess with inflammatory adhesions to the urinary bladder, ureter and ductus deferens.
**Follow-up:** 2 months, no signs of disease recurrence.

The large histologic section in Figure 5.**8** demonstrates a complex picture. Centrally, corresponding to the red-colored area in Figure 5.**8 e**, a large diverticle showing deep ulceration in the mucosa is seen. The mucosa also shows signs of active inflammation. As an illustration of this process, a cryptal abscess is demonstrated in Figure 5.**8 a**. Around the lumen of the diverticle, an intensive inflammatory reaction, forming a peridiverticular abscess, is seen. As a consequence of the inflammatory reaction, fibrous adhesions have developed. The operation was widened to include a segment of the ureter (marked with the red rectangle in the schematic image, Fig. 5.**8 e** and microscopically magnified in Fig. 5.**8 b**), a segment of the ductus deferens (marked with the blue rectangle and magnified in Fig. 5.**8 c**), and a part of the wall of the urinary bladder (marked with the orange rectangle and magnified in Fig. 5.**8 d**). The complex pseudopolypous silhouette of the mucosa is well seen in the large section (two of the pseudopolyps are indicated with the blue arrows in the schematic image). Several enlarged lymph nodes were also present in the specimen (indicated with the yellow arrows in Fig. 5.**8 e**). The green arrow in the figure marks another diverticle.

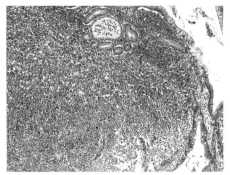

Fig. 5.**8 a**

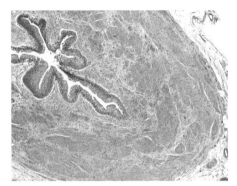

Fig. 5.**8 b**

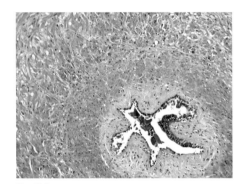

Fig. 5.**8 c**

### Practical points

- A single large section may include transection of different organs, while at the same time demonstrating their relation in the pathological process.

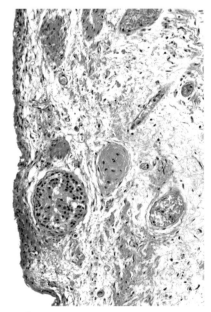

Fig. 5.**8 d**

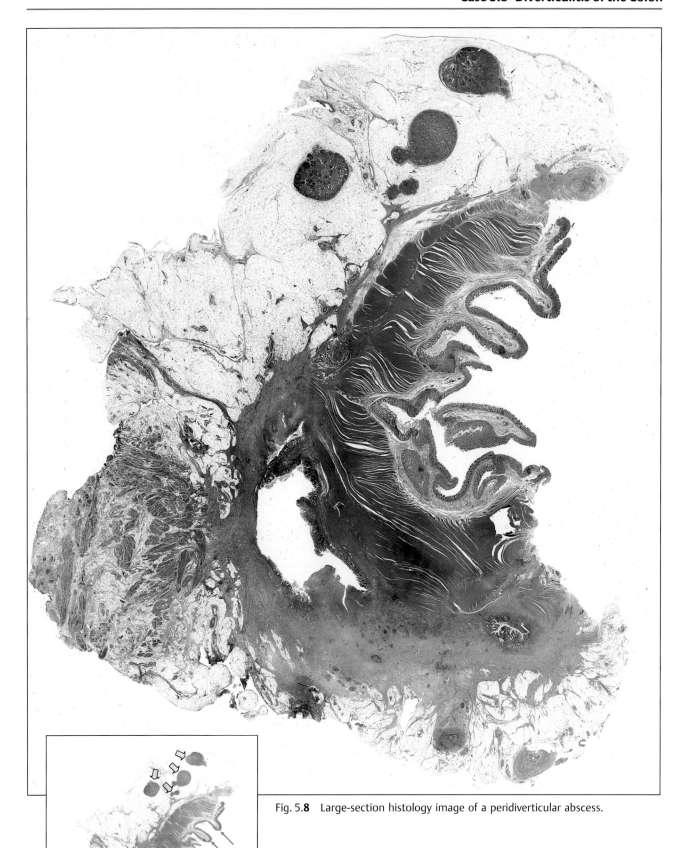

Fig. 5.**8** Large-section histology image of a peridiverticular abscess.

Fig. 5.**8 e** Schematic guide to the morphologic details in the large section in Fig. 5.**8**.

## Case 5.9 Hemorrhagic Infarction of the Small Intestine

**Patient data:** 73-year-old man presenting with acute abdominal pain and signs of peritonitis.
**Surgical treatment:** Resection of an ileal segment, no pre-operative treatment.
**Specimen:** 38-cm-long segment of the small intestine centrally, with a red- to blue-colored infarcted area and containing necrotic-hemorrhagic debris.
**Histopathologic diagnosis:** Hemorrhagic infarction of the small intestine due to mesenterial thrombosis. Local peritonitis. No malignancy.
**Follow-up:** Died of heart failure 15 months after the operation.

The large histologic section demonstrated in Figure 5.**9** was taken through a part of the small intestine, which showed signs of hemorrhagic infarction after mesenterial thrombosis. It demonstrates the attenuated and partly ulcerated mucosa, and the edema and hemorrhage in the intestinal wall as well as in the mesenterium. Figure 5.**9 a**, **b** represents magnified details of the infarcted intestinal wall (corresponding to the area of the yellow and the green rectangle in the schematic image, Fig. 5.**9 d**, respectively). Figure 5.**9 c** demonstrates a magnified image of the lymph node in the mesenterium (marked with the red circle in Fig. 5.**9 d**) showing signs of recent hemorrhage.

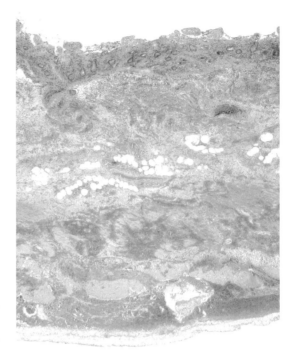

Fig. 5.**9 a**

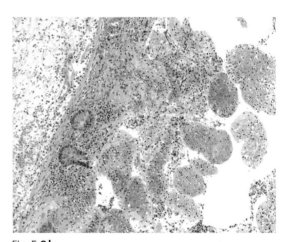

Fig. 5.**9 b**

### Practical points

- The large histologic sections include the transsection of the intestinal wall together with the structures of the mesentery, facilitating the evaluation of the pathologic changes in all these structures at the same time.

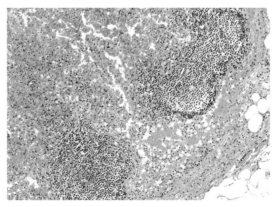

Fig. 5.**9 c**

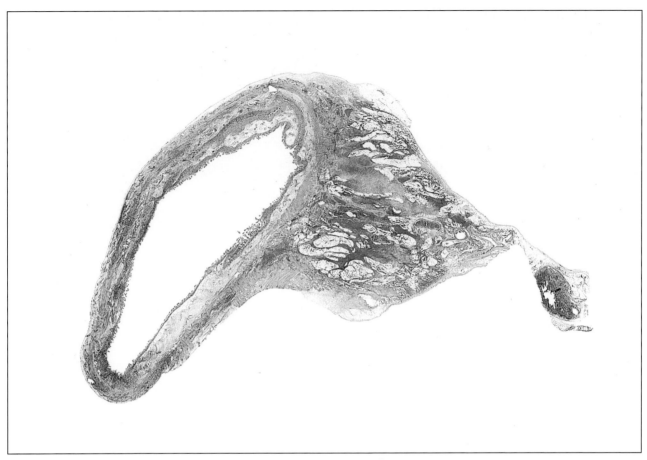

Fig. 5.**9**  Large-section histology image of hemorrhagic infarction of the small intestine.

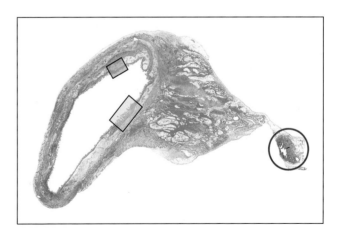

Fig. 5.**9 d**  Schematic guide to the morphologic details in the large section in Fig. 5.**9**.

## Case 5.10 Intestinal Endometriosis

**Patient data:** 31-year-old woman presenting with abdominal pain and operated on because of a tumor-like lesion in the ileocecal region.
**Surgical treatment:** Ileocecal resection, no preoperative treatment.
**Specimen:** 20-cm-long segment of the large intestine together with a 4-cm part of the terminal ileum and inverted appendix. A 6-cm tumor-like mass with small blood-filled spaces on the cut surface was present in the ileocecal area.
**Histopathologic diagnosis:** Intestinal endometriosis. No malignancy
**Follow-up:** 17 months, no signs of disease recurrence.

This young woman was operated on because of a suspicious mass in the ileocoecal region causing intestinal subobstruction. The large section in Figure 5.**10** demonstrates a part of the wall of the terminal ileum (the surface of the ileal mucosa is indicated with blue arrows in the schematic image, Fig. 5.**10 d**) as well as the wall of the cecum (indicated with orange arrows in the schematic image). A thickening of the muscular layer in the interface of the two intestinal loops is very well seen. Histologic examination revealed foci of endometriosis with typical stroma and endometrioid glands, as illustrated in Figure 5.**10 a** (corresponding to the area of the red rectangle in Fig. 5.**10 d**). Some of the foci of the endometriosis showed signs of recent bleeding (Fig. 5.**10 b**, corresponding to the area of the blue rectangle). Figure 5.**10 c** is a magnified image of a focus of endometriosis. Note the Payer's plaque in the upper part of the intestinal mucosa in the large-section image (indicated with the middle blue arrow in Fig. 5.**10 d**).

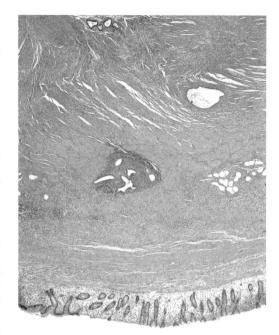

Fig. 5.**10 a**

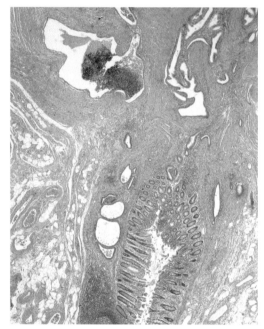

Fig. 5.**10 b**

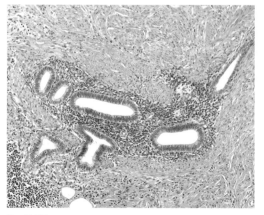

**Practical points**

- The large section images are not only superior to the traditional technique in terms of diagnostic values, but also in terms of aesthetics.

Fig. 5.**10 c**

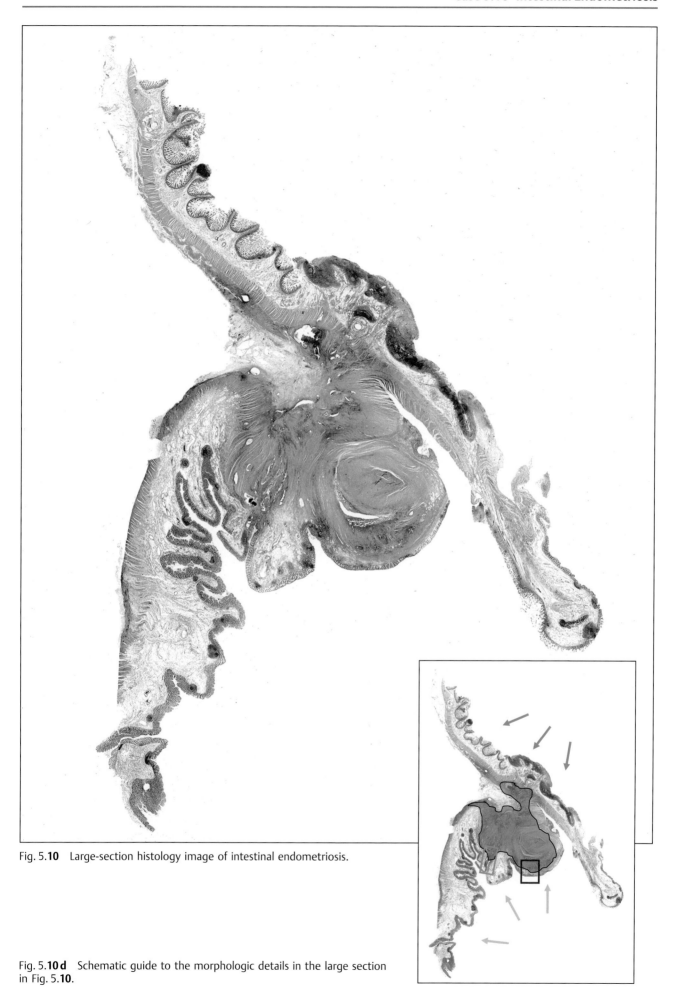

Fig. 5.**10**   Large-section histology image of intestinal endometriosis.

Fig. 5.**10 d**   Schematic guide to the morphologic details in the large section in Fig. 5.**10**.

# 6 Technical Considerations

Proper orientation and cut-up of the surgical specimen is essential in obtaining representative large sections. In the ideal situation, the rectal amputates (Fig. 6.1) or other colorectal resection preparations are first cleaned and filled with fixative, closed by sutures or clips at both ends, and then immersed in the proper amount of fixative in a container larger than the specimen. This procedure offers optimal fixation of the tissue, both in the inner and outer layers of the intestine. If the fixation is carried out only by immersing the specimen in a small amount of formalin, autolytic changes takes place that disturb the microscopic evaluation. This may also be prevented if the specimen is opened longitudinally on its front side. Cutting through the lesions or distorting them by forcing the specimen into an inappropriately small container should be avoided as it may substantially influence the macroscopic and subgross appearance of the lesion, sometimes making correlation of the large-section image with the original endoscopic image impossible.

Close inspection of the specimen, especially of the frontal (Fig. 6.2) and the mesorectal (Fig. 6.3) surfaces, helps the pathologist in planning the dissection. Macroscopically seen tumor tissue on these surfaces has to be histologically documented, one of the advantages of large sections. Clinical information about the position of the tumor within the specimen is also helpful as it directs the attention of the pathologist to the most important part of the specimen. We recommend serial sectioning of the specimen perpendicular to the longitudinal axis (demonstrated in Figs. 6.4–6.7). The slices must be 3- to 5-mm thick to allow proper dehydration and further laboratory processing. This thickness is relatively easy to achieve if the specimen is properly fixed and if a sharp instrument with a disposable blade is used. Cutting up the specimen without prior fixation may reduce laboratory turnover time for this type of preparation, but it requires substantial experience.

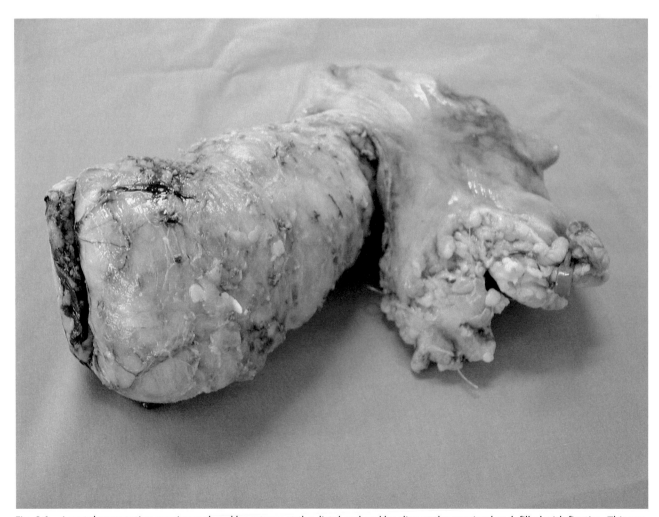

Fig. 6.1  A rectal amputation specimen closed by sutures at the distal end and by clips at the proximal end, filled with fixative. This procedure assures proper preservation of the histologic details.

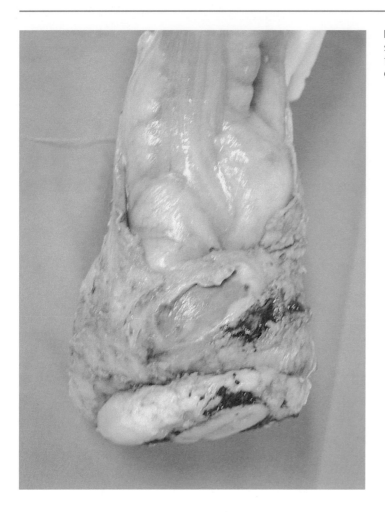

Fig. 6.**2** The ventral, partly peritonealized, anatomic surface of the rectal specimen. The presence of peritoneum on this surface guides the pathologist in proper orientation of the specimen.

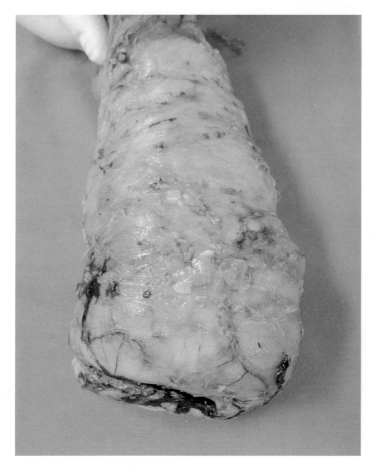

Fig. 6.**3** The mesorectal surface of the specimen shown in Fig. 6.**2**. This surface is artificial, produced by surgery. Proper visualization of this surface in the large section is essential for evaluation of the result and quality of the surgical intervention.

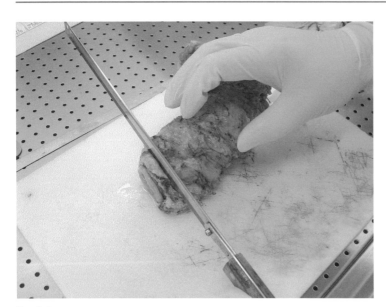

Figs. 6.**4**–6.**6** Serial slicing of the specimen perpendicular to the longitudinal axis. A knife with a very sharp disposable blade is needed for producing evenly thick 3–5-mm slices.

Fig. 6.**4**

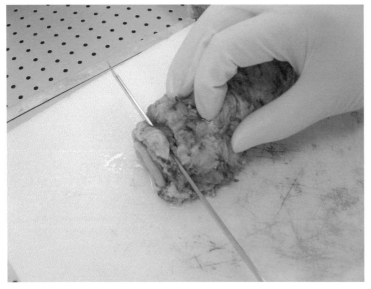

Fig. 6.**5**

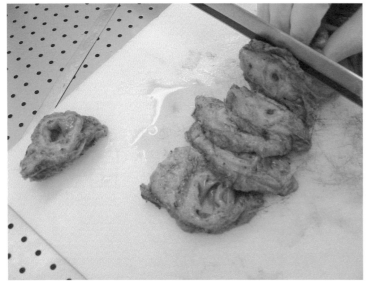

Fig. 6.**6**

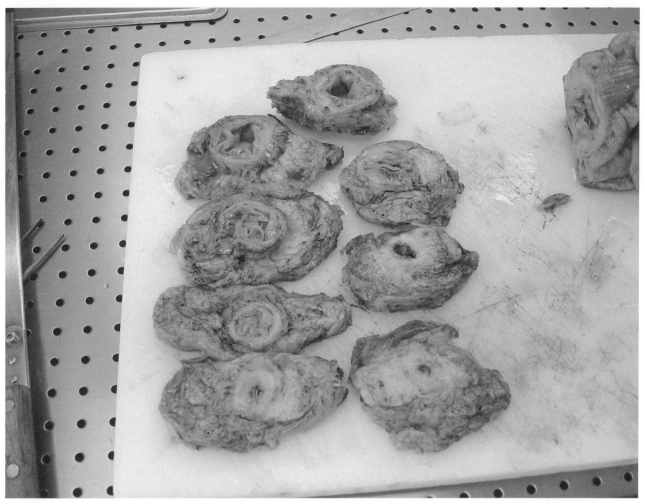

Fig. 6.**7** The serial slicing of the specimen illustrated in the previous figures provides an accurate, ordered display of all grossly detectable lesions within the specimen.

A thorough naked-eye examination of the sections, especially of the cut surfaces, is essential in choosing the proper slice for embedding. The pathologist should find the slice with the deepest level of invasion. Additional slices with abnormalities not seen in the slice with the deepest invasion are also selected for embedding. The slices should be palpated since palpation and macroscopic examination of the pericolic-perirectal fatty tissue are necessary in order to find all the lymph nodes.

The selected tissue slices are stretched on a cork plate and pinned, with the surface to be cut facing down (Figs. 6.**8**–6.**11**). The slices are immersed in dishes containing standard formalin solution for tissue fixation (Fig. 6.**11**). If the specimen was already properly fixed before slicing, the fixation time of the slice is reduced to 2–5 h. If the specimen was sliced unfixed, the fixation time for the slice is 12–24 h. By fixing the tissue when it is stretched, a fairly flat surface can be achieved. Thorough fixation of the slices is essential in this technique. Microwave treatment can considerably reduce the time necessary for optimal fixation.

After fixation, the slices are removed from the cork plate and placed into special-sized containers in an automatic tissue processor (Figs. 6.**12** and 6.**13**). Before processing, slices that are already fixed can be trimmed to obtain the ideal thickness of 3–4 mm throughout the entire slice.

Formation of large paraffin blocks for embedding of the slices is demonstrated in Figures 6.**14**–6.**19**. The size of the block can be slightly modified depending on the size of the tissue slice.

Sectioning of the large blocks is carried out using a special macrotome (Figs. 6.**20** and 6.**21**). The most important factor in obtaining large histologic sections of proper quality is a skillful and experienced technician (Figs. 6.**22**–6.**26**).

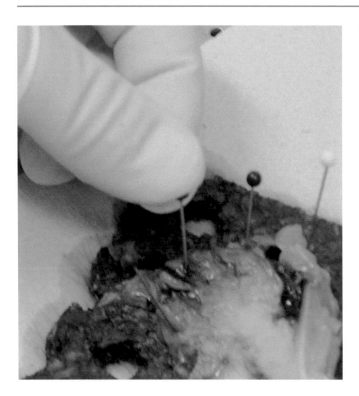

Fig. 6.**8** For additional fixation the selected slice(s) is stretched over a cork plate and pinned.

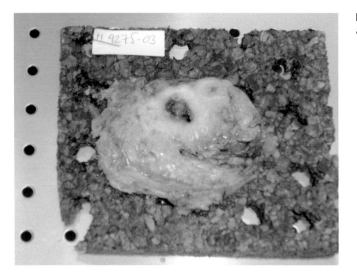

Fig. 6.**9** The procedure allows proper fixation and assures an evenly flat cut-surface (facing down).

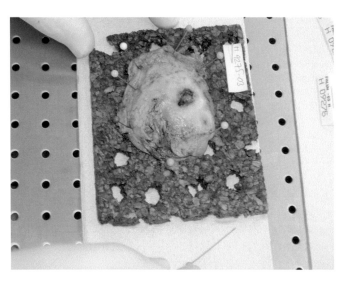

Fig. 6.**10** Marking the slices properly with the patient data is mandatory. Marking dyes may also be used to maintain the orientation of the slice during the laboratory work-up.

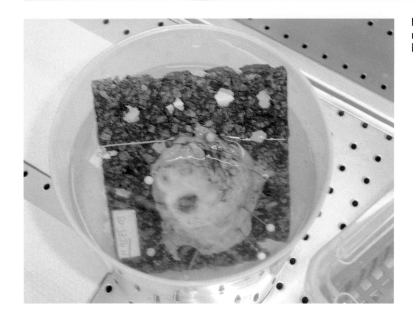

Fig. 6.**11**   A tissue slice on a cork plate is immersed in a dish containing standard formalin solution for tissue fixation.

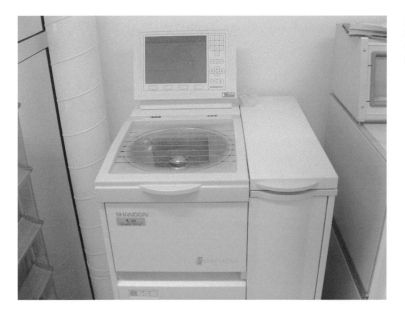

Fig. 6.**12**   Processing (dehydration) of the tissue slice is essentially the same as for the traditional small tissue samples and can be carried out in any commercially available automatic processor.

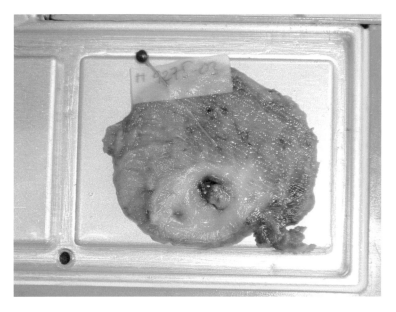

Fig. 6.**13**   The processed tissue slice, containing paraffin.

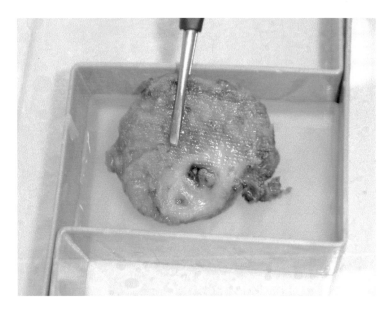

Fig. 6.**14** Metal brackets can be used to make the paraffin blocks, as demonstrated in this image. By changing the distance between the brackets one can adjust the size of the paraffin block to the size of the tissue slice. The temperature of the underlying glass plate leads to relatively rapid cooling and hardening of the liquid paraffin, keeping the rest of the warm paraffin within the bracketed space.

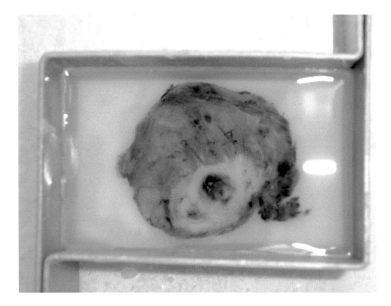

Fig. 6.**15** The processed tissue slice is immersed in the liquid paraffin.

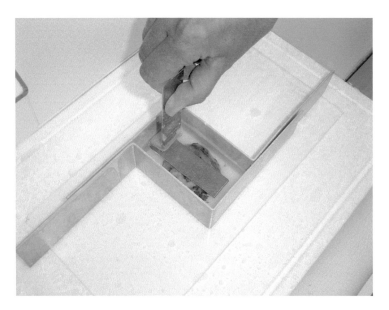

Fig. 6.**16** To help achieve an evenly flat cut surface (facing down), the slice is pushed against the bottom of the space.

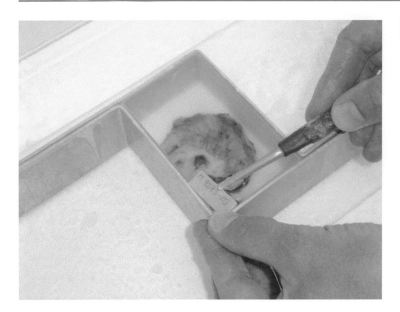

Fig. 6.**17** Marking of the paraffin block with a serial number.

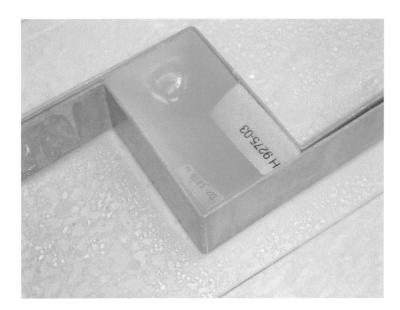

Fig. 6.**18** The liquid paraffin takes several hours to cool and stiffen at normal room temperature.

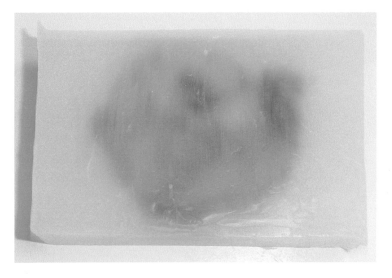

Fig. 6.**19** The lower surface of the large paraffin block, ready to be cut in the macrotome. The blocks are stored in a refrigerator (4 °C) before cutting.

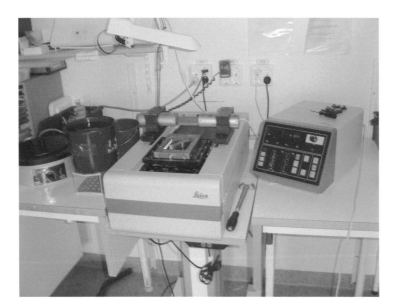

Fig. 6.**20** An automated macrotome, specially designed to cut large paraffin blocks.

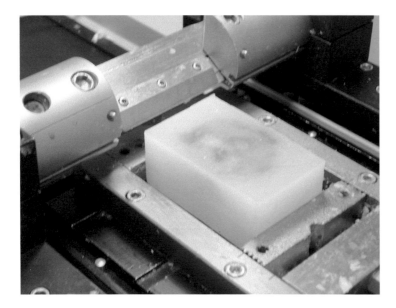

Fig. 6.**21** The macrotome differs from a routine microtome used in pathology laboratories in the size of the block holder and in the width of the cutting blade.

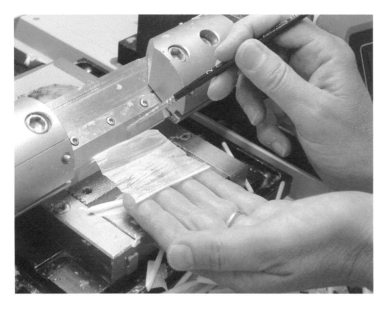

Fig. 6.**22** The most important factor in obtaining the uniformly thin (3–4 microns) large paraffin section is the skilful and specially trained laboratory technician.

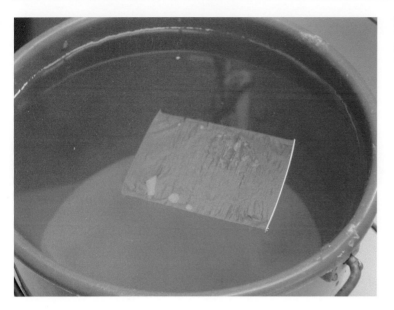

Fig. 6.**23**   The thin section of paraffin-embedded tissue is initially wrinkled. It is evenly smoothed out in cold and warm water baths. The first step, a cold water bath, is illustrated in this figure.

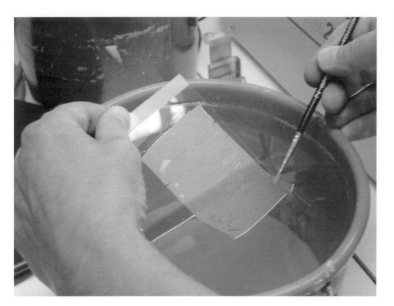

Fig. 6.**24**   The section is caught on a glass slide; its position is carefully adjusted.

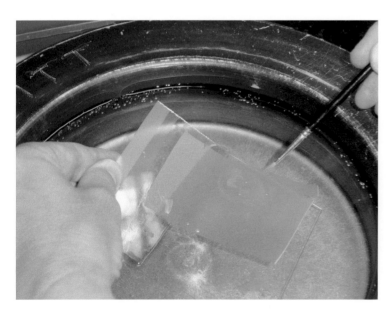

Fig. 6.**25**   The temperature of the warm water bath facilitates smoothing out of the section on the glass slide.

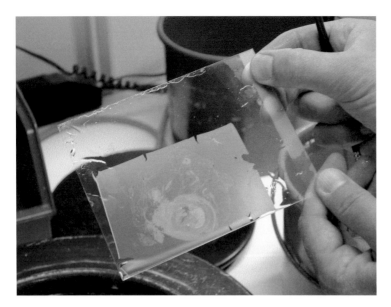

Fig. 6.**26** The resulting smoothed-out large block paraffin section on the glass slide. The section has to be deparaffinized in a thermostat before staining.

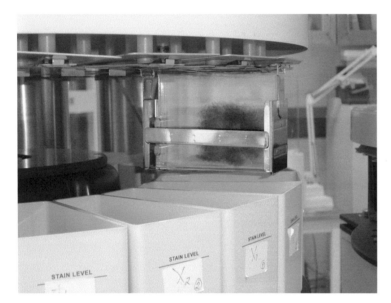

Fig. 6.**27** Staining can be performed in any commercially available automated stainer if modified holders adjusted to the size of the large glass slide are used. The staining program for any routine staining is the same as for the traditional small sections.

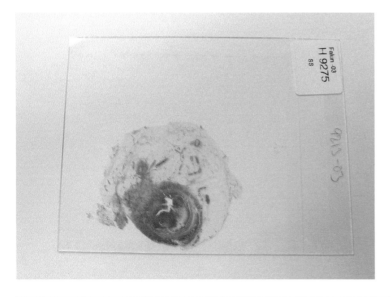

Fig. 6.**28** The stained large histologic section is mounted as usual and covered by a large-sized cover slide. We use commercially available standard-sized object glass (90 × 120 mm) and corresponding cover slide in our laboratory.

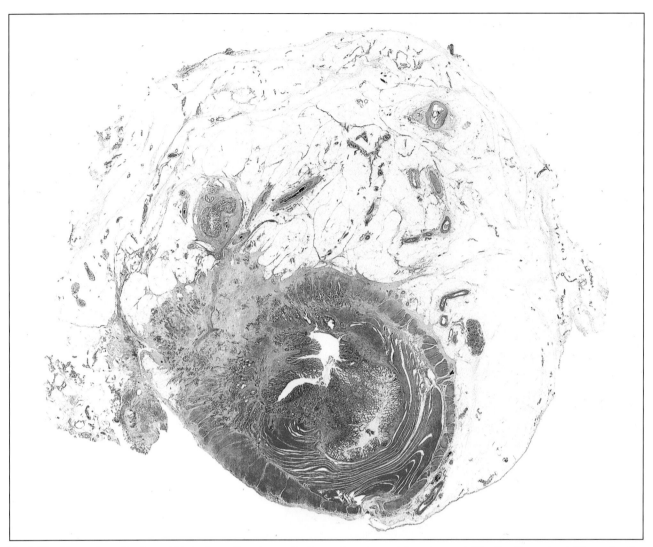

Fig. 6.**29**   The end result: a large histologic section demonstrating an invasive rectal carcinoma infiltrating the perirectal tissue (on the left side of the image). Note a diverticle, several blood vessels, and a lymph node in the mesorectum.

For staining large histologic sections, we use modified holders that are placed into the automatic stainer, also used routinely for small blocks (Fig. 6.**27**). The recipe for hematoxylin and eosin staining is the same as that for conventional histologic sections. A properly processed large section has a thickness of 3–4 µm, and has the same staining characteristics, the same preservation of cellular details, and the same overall quality as conventional small block sections (Figs. 6.**28** and 6.**29**).

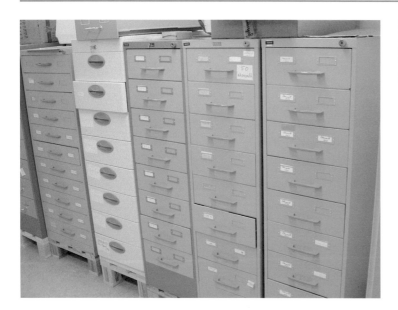

Fig. 6.**30** File cabinets designed for the storage of large histologic slides. It is important that the slides are perfectly dry before they are put in this archive. The drying process at room temperature may take several weeks.

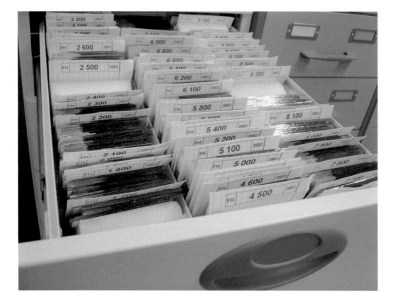

Fig. 6.**31** Large histologic sections archived in order of their laboratory serial number.

Large histologic sections can be easily archived and storaged (Figs. 6.**30** and 6.**31**). The four file cabinets shown in Figure 6.**30** contain the large sections produced in our department from 1986 to 2003, corresponding to about 5600 different cases. Identification of these cases is similar to the archiving of conventional small histologic slides.

Large histologic sections are regularly used in clinicopathological conferences, tumor boards, and other meetings in our institution. A simple overhead projection of the large section gives a magnified image with superior resolution quality. Transection of the tumor, its relation to normal structures, the circumferential margin, several lymph nodes, and other details are easily demonstrated. The projected image directly correlates with endoscopic and macroscopic findings. In addition, it is fully accepted by clinicians for discussing most of the clinically relevant questions related to the completeness of the surgical intervention, depth of tumor infiltration, the presence or absence of macrometastases, etc. If histological details need to demonstrated, the same large section can be viewed under the microscope.

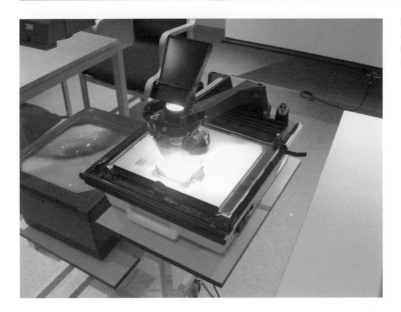

Fig. 6.**32**  A specially designed (commercially available) overhead projector used in our conference room for projecting the archived large-section slides.

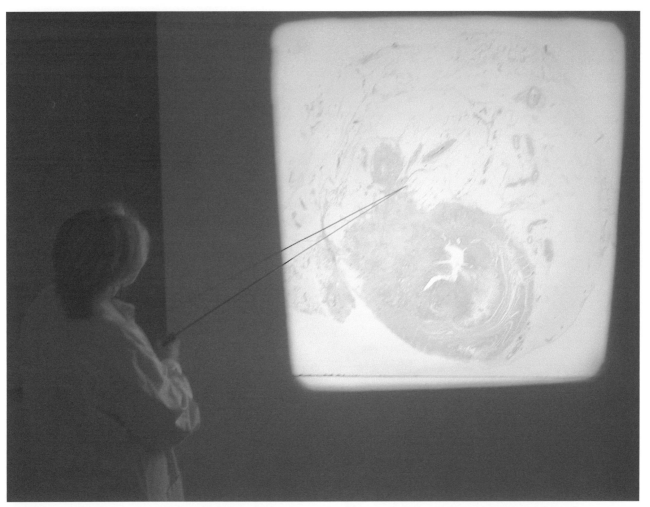

Fig. 6.**33**  The projected image is of superior quality with sufficient subgross details for successful communication between the pathologist and the clinicians.

# References

AJCC. Cancer staging handbook. TNM classification of malignant tumours. 6th edn. Springer, New York, Berlin, Heidelberg, Barcelona, Hong Kong, London, Milan, Paris, Singapore, Tokyo, 2002

Cecil TD et al. Total mesorectal excision results in low local recurrence rates in lymph node-positive rectal cancer. Dis Colon Rectum 2004;47:1145–50.

Dukes CE. Cancer of the rectum: analysis of 1000 cases. J Pathol Bacteiol 1940;50:527–39.

Heald RJ, Ryall RDH. Recurrence and survival after total mesorectal excision of the rectal cancer. Lancet 1986;1:1479.82.

Jackson PA et al. A comparison of large block macrosectioning and conventional techniques in breast pathology. Virchows Archiv 1994;425:243–8.

Koh DM et al. Rectal cancer: mesorectal lymph nodes at MR imaging with USPIO versus histopathologic findings – initial observations. Radiology 2004;231:91–9.

Leong AF. Total mesorectal excision (TME) – twenty years on. Ann Acad Med Singapore 2003;32:159–62.

Nagtegaal ID et al. Circumferential margin involvement is still an important predictor of local recurrence in rectal carcinoma. Am J Surg Pathol 2003;26(3):350–7.

Nakayama H et al. Papillary adenocarcinoma of the sigmoid colon associated with psammoma bodies and hyaline globules: report of a case. Jpn J Clin Oncol 1997;27:193–6.

Nasir A et al. Flat and polypoid adenocarcinomas of the colorectum: a comparative histomorphologic analysis of 47 cases.Hum Pathol 2004;35:604–11.

Parkin D et al. Cancer incidence in five continents, VI. IARC, Lyon, 1992.

Spark RP. Filiform polyposis of the colon. First report in a case of transmural colitis (Crohn's disease). Am J Dig Dis 1976;21(9):809–14.

Tot T, Tabár L, Dean PB. The pressing need for better histologic-mammographic correlation of the many variations in normal breast anatomy. Virchows Arch 2000;437:338–44.

Tot T. The diffuse type of invasive lobular carcinoma of the breast: morphology and prognosis. Virchows Arch 2000;443(6):718–24

Tot T, Tabár L, Dean PB. Practical breast pathology, Chapter 8 The postoperative work-up. Thieme Stuttgart, New York, pp 115–23, 2002

Tot T. Cytokeratins 20 and 7 as biomarkers: usefulness in discriminating primary from metastatic adenocarcinoma. Eur J Cancer 2002;38; 758–63.

Tot T. Identifying colorectal metastases in liver biopsies: the novel CDX2 antibody is less specific than the cytokeratin 20+/7- phenotype. Med Sci Monit 2004;10; BR139–43.

Wei JT et al. Quality of colon carcinoma pathology reporting. A process of care study. Cancer2004;100;1263–7.

Winther KV et al. Screening for dysplasia and TP53 mutations in closed rectal stump of patients with ulcerative colitis and Crohn disease. Scand J Gastroenterol 2004;39; 232–7.

# Index